Super Duper® Publications

"Say & Do®"
Artic Reps

124 Reproducible Artic Sheets for S, R, L, Blends, SH, CH, F, G, K

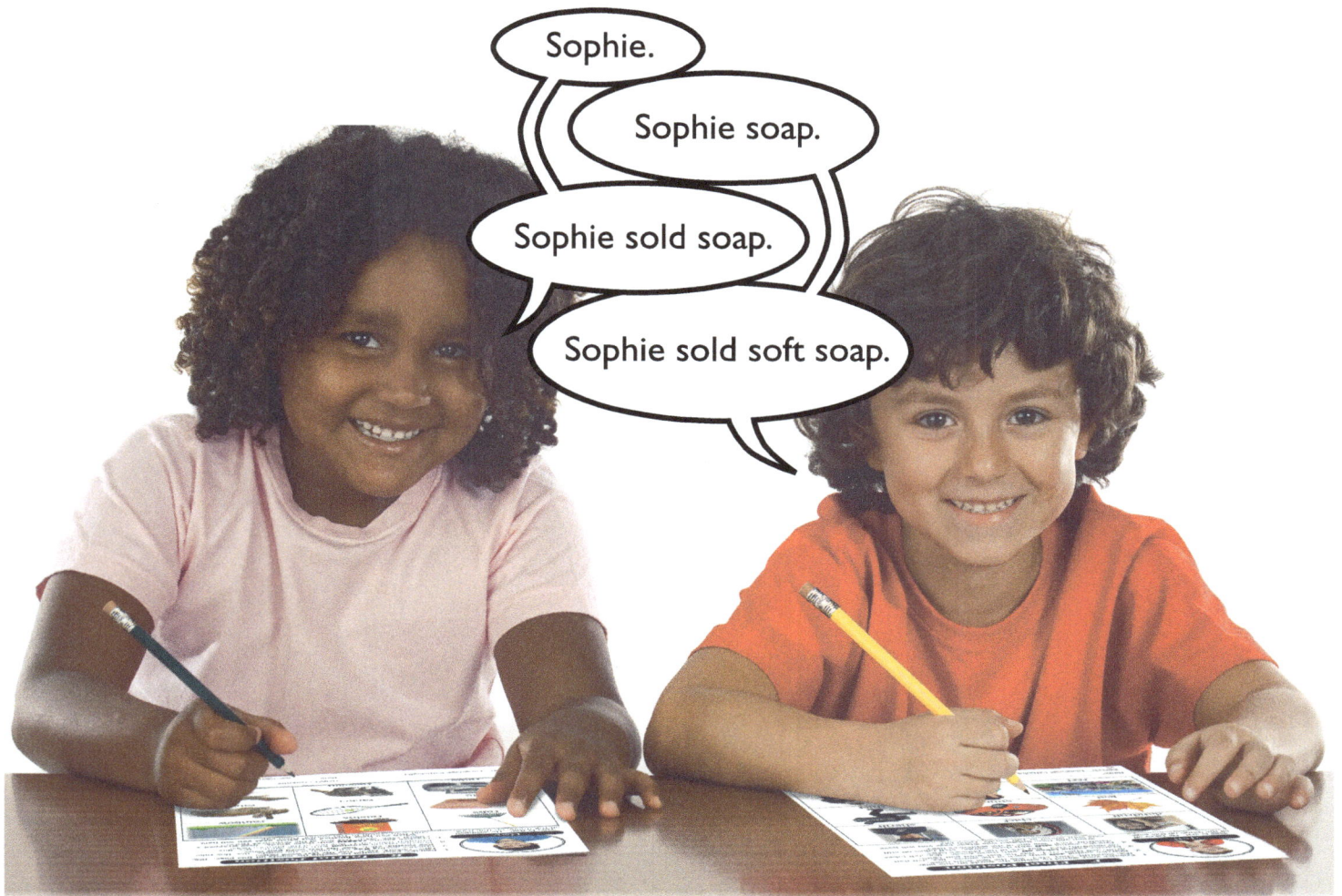

Sophie.

Sophie soap.

Sophie sold soap.

Sophie sold soft soap.

Written by Bonnie O'Bryan
Photography by Thinkstock® and Super Duper® Staff

**Photos ©2015
Super Duper® and Thinkstock®**

Printed in the United States

ISBN 978-1-58650-075-7

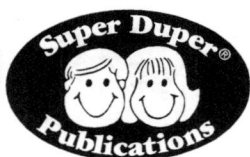

**Super Duper® Publications
www.superduperinc.com
1-800-277-8737**

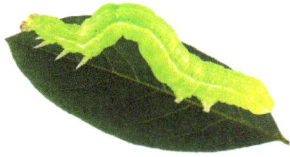

Say & Do® Artic Reps

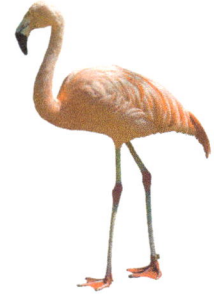

Say & Do® Artic Reps is an articulation strengthening and reinforcement program. Originally developed for the Cleveland Public Schools Speech Language Services, *Say & Do® Artic Reps* is for the primary or non-reading child diagnosed with articulation problems. *Say & Do® Artic Reps* specifically addresses the S, R, L, Blends, SH, CH, F, G and K phonemes.

Say & Do® Artic Reps helps the child improve articulation skills by repetition – "reps" – of the target sound in words, word pairs, sentences and expanded sentences. Phonemes are presented in the beginning, medial and final positions. The photos add a level of fun and visual cueing for early learners. Students will enjoy the colorful photos and silly sentences.

This manual includes an explanation of the program, home directions, Artic Reps photo pages, and a tracking sheet. The tracking sheet provides a means for the therapist and child to have a log of responses, keeping the therapist and child aware of her/his level of progress in the program. This is also a simple and efficient way to keep information for documentation. Keep the sheet in a folder. At the beginning of the session, the therapist/child can identify which step of the program she/he is working on. The therapist/child may use a clicker to identify mistakes. Since the number of correct responses is set in advance, the therapist and child can easily keep track of the number of correct responses.

These photo pages may be copied on colored card stock for easy sound identification (ex: R-Red, L-Yellow, S-White, etc.). Pages may be laminated for long-lasting use. Also, the therapist may copy the pages and send them home with the child along with the Home Program Explanation.

Use the Artic Reps program to reinforce phonological work or to establish and reinforce language work. Use the photos and words for vocabulary development; sentence structure work with pronouns, verbs, and adjectives; and a variety of activities as determined by the therapist. I hope all who use this program find it as valuable as I have. My students and I have enjoyed it immensely.

— *Bonnie O'Bryan*

Table of Contents

#BKCD-273 • *See It! Say It! Artic Reps* • ©2015 Super Duper® Publications • www.superduperinc.com

Artic Picture Reps Program

Say & Do® Artic Reps is an articulation strengthening program designed for the primary or non-reading student with articulation errors. Each page presents 9 photos addressing these sounds – SH, CH, F, G, K, S, R, L, and Blends. *Say & Do® Artic Reps* progresses by sound position through repetitions – "reps" – of words, word pairs, sentences, and expanded sentences. There are multiple photo pages per target sound with 100 "reps" per page. "Reps" help stabilize good sound production and promotes carryover.

An explanation of the therapy program, the home program and the tracking sheet follow.

Therapy Program

The following "Initial S" page (p. 117) illustrates how the program works.

Sophie

S – Initial Position

This is Sophie. She sold all the things on this page.

1. Practice your sound by saying the words on this page. (Ex. soap, sock, etc.). Say the last word twice.
2. Practice saying **Sophie** with each of the words. (Ex. Sophie soap, Sophie sock, etc.). Say the last word pair twice.
3. Practice saying **sold** with these words. (Ex. Sophie sold soap, etc.). Say one of the phrases twice.
4. Practice saying **soft** with these words. (Sophie sold soft soap, etc.). Say one of the sentences twice.

When you have finished this whole page you will have said your sound in 100 words! Good job!

soap	sock	soda
soup	soccer ball	sofa
soil	swordfish	sword

Name _____   Helper Signature _____

Speech - Language Pathologist _____   Date _____

#BK-273 • *Say & Do® Artic Reps* • ©2015 Super Duper® Publications • www.superduperinc.com   117

Please note that since this program begins at the word level, it assumes correction of the target phoneme has already taken place.

Each Photo Rep page has a character (the "Repper") in the upper left hand corner of the page. Here the Repper is Sophie. Before beginning the steps below, the student says the Repper's name ("Sophie"). The child then follows the directions on the page in sequential order.

(1)   Words – Have the child say each word on the page once, except the last word, which he/she should say twice (soap, sock, soda, etc.). This totals 10 "Initial S" reps. If the child says 9 out of 10 words correctly, proceed to (#2) Word Pairs.

(2)   Word Pairs – Have the child say the Repper's name followed by the word in each photo (Sophie - soap; Sophie - sock; Sophie - soda; etc.) The child says the last word pair twice. This totals 20 more "Initial S" reps. If the child says 18 or more word pairs correctly, proceed to (#3) Phrases.

(3)   Sentences – Have the child say the Repper's name, the action word in bold type, and the photo words in sentences. (Sophie sold soap; Sophie sold sock; Sophie sold soda; etc.). Sometimes you must add an "a" or "the" to the sentence for it to be grammactically correct. Have the child repeat the last sentence (Sophie sold sword) twice. This totals 30 more reps. If the child says 27 or more sentences correctly, proceed to (#4) Expanded Sentences.

(4)   Expanded Sentences – Have the child say the Repper's name, the action word, the describing word in bold type, and the picture word in expanded sentences (Sophie sold soft soap; Sophie sold a soft sock; etc.). Sometimes you must add an "a" or "the" to the sentence for it to be grammatically correct. Have the student say the last expanded sentence twice. (Sophie sold a soft sword.) This totals 40 more reps. If the child says 36 or more sentences correctly, you may proceed to any carryover activities you choose (Ex: Have the child tell you more about one or more of the sentences.)

Some of the word pairs and/or sentences may be silly, or even nonsensical. This is okay! The main objective of the program is to have the child practice his/her target phoneme as many times as possible.

When the child successfully completes a page, he/she has said the target sound correctly in 100 words.

Home Program

The Artic Photo Reps program is ideal for home practice and reinforcement. Attach a Parent/Helper Letter with practice instructions to the Photo Reps pages and send home.

Tracking Sheet

A tracking sheet to record student progress appears on page x. A student should complete at least 90% of each step correctly before moving to the next step. (9/10, 18/20, 27/30, 36/40) The tracking sheet gives the student a record of success and progression. It also provides the SLP with IEP, lesson plan, and document information.

After a student finishes all steps of the program, use the photos for carryover work. Have your student tell a story about one of the sentences. Use *Say & Do® Artic Reps* for reinforcement of phonological and language work. Be creative and have fun with *Say & Do® Artic Reps*!!

Picture pages may be copied on colored stock and laminated for in-session use. They can also be copied individually or in a unit for home assignments.

#BKCD-273 • *See It! Say It! Artic Reps* • ©2015 Super Duper® Publications • www.superduperinc.com

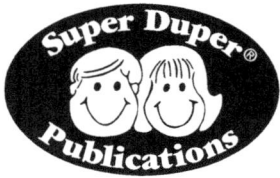

Date _____

Dear Parent/Helper:

Your child is learning to say his/her sound correctly in the _____ position(s). Attached to this letter is an Artic Reps home practice sheet. The activities on this sheet are simple, and they will help your child learn to say his/her target sound correctly through lots of repetition.

Here's how it works! The person in the upper left-hand corner of the page is a "Repper." Have your child say the Repper's name. Next, have your child complete the repetition activities in the boxes checked below.

❑ Step 1 only   <u>Words</u> – Have your child say each photo word on the page one time and say the last word twice.

❑ Steps 1 and 2 only   <u>Word Pairs</u> – After completing Step 1, have your child say the Repper's name with each photo word. Repeat the last word pair twice.

❑ Steps 1, 2 & 3   <u>Sentences</u> – After completing Steps 1 & 2, have your child say the Repper's name, the action word (in bold type), and the photo word once. Repeat the last sentence twice.

❑ Steps 1, 2, 3 & 4   <u>Expanded Sentences</u> – After completing Steps 1, 2 & 3, have your child say the Repper's name, the action word, the bold describing word, and the photo words in sentences. Repeat the last sentence twice. Some of the sentences will be silly. That is okay! The idea is to get lots of practice.

_____

_____

_____

After you complete these activities with your child, please sign this sheet below and have your child return it to me by _____.

Thanks for your help!

_____   _____
Speech-Language Pathologist   Parent Signature

Say & Do® Artic Reps Tracking Sheet

Name _____   Sound _____

Position _____

Date   Correct Responses/ Total Responses

_____   ❑ words   ___/10   ___/10   ___/10   ___/10
                 ❑ word pairs   ___/20   ___/20   ___/20   ___/20
                 ❑ sentences   ___/30   ___/30   ___/30   ___/30
                 ❑ expanded   ___/40   ___/40   ___/40   ___/40
                   sentences

Date   Correct Responses/ Total Responses

_____   ❑ words   ___/10   ___/10   ___/10   ___/10
                 ❑ word pairs   ___/20   ___/20   ___/20   ___/20
                 ❑ sentences   ___/30   ___/30   ___/30   ___/30
                 ❑ expanded   ___/40   ___/40   ___/40   ___/40
                   sentences

Date   Correct Responses/ Total Responses

_____   ❑ words   ___/10   ___/10   ___/10   ___/10
                 ❑ word pairs   ___/20   ___/20   ___/20   ___/20
                 ❑ sentences   ___/30   ___/30   ___/30   ___/30
                 ❑ expanded   ___/40   ___/40   ___/40   ___/40
                   sentences

Date   Correct Responses/ Total Responses

_____   ❑ words   ___/10   ___/10   ___/10   ___/10
                 ❑ word pairs   ___/20   ___/20   ___/20   ___/20
                 ❑ sentences   ___/30   ___/30   ___/30   ___/30
                 ❑ expanded   ___/40   ___/40   ___/40   ___/40
                   sentences

Date   Correct Responses/ Total Responses

_____   ❑ words   ___/10   ___/10   ___/10   ___/10
                 ❑ word pairs   ___/20   ___/20   ___/20   ___/20
                 ❑ sentences   ___/30   ___/30   ___/30   ___/30
                 ❑ expanded   ___/40   ___/40   ___/40   ___/40
                   sentences

#BKCD-273 • *See It! Say It! Artic Reps* • ©2015 Super Duper® Publications • www.superduperinc.com

CH

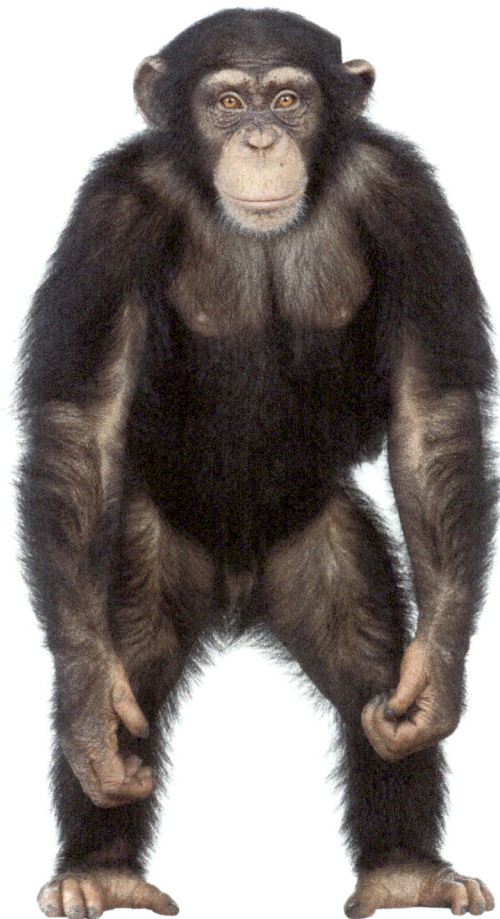

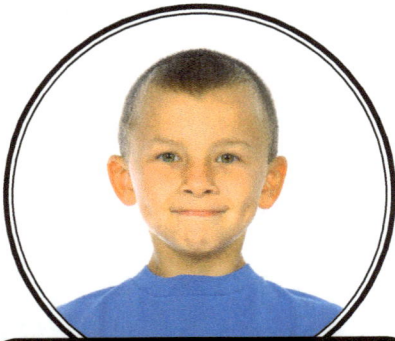

Chad

This is Chad. He chased all the things on this page.

CH – Initial Position

1. Practice your sound by saying the words on this page. (Ex. Charles, change, etc.). Say the last word twice.

2. Practice saying **Chad** with each of the words. (Ex. Chad Charles, Chad change, etc.). Say the last word pair twice.

3. Practice saying **chased** with these words. (Ex. Chad chased Charles, etc.). Say one of the sentences twice.

4. Practice saying **charming** with these words. (Chad chased the charming Charles, etc.). Say one of the expanded sentences twice.

When you finish this whole page, you will have said your sound in 100 words! Good job!

Charles	change	chairman
challenger	champ	chariot
chain	charge cards	chatter box

Name _____

Helper Signature _____

Speech - Language Pathologist _____

Date _____

#BKCD-273 • Say & Do® Artic Reps • ©2015 Super Duper® Publications • www.superduperinc.com

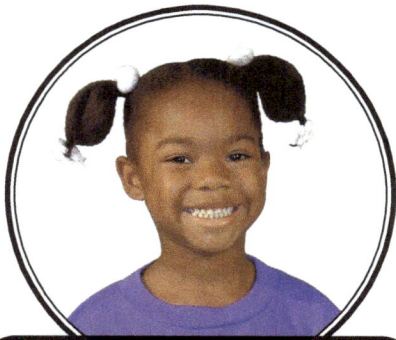

Chelsea

This is Chelsea. She chewed all the things on this page.

CH – Initial Position

1. Practice your sound by saying the words on this page. (Ex. checkbook, cherries, etc.). Say the last word twice.
2. Practice saying **Chelsea** with each of the words. (Ex. Chelsea checkbook, Chelsea cherries, etc.). Say the last word pair twice.
3. Practice saying **chewed** with these words. (Ex. Chelsea chewed a checkbook, etc.). Say one of the sentences twice.
4. Practice saying **cheap** with these words. (Chelsea chewed a cheap checkbook, etc.). Say one of the expanded sentences twice.

When you finish this whole page, you will have said your sound in 100 words! Good job!

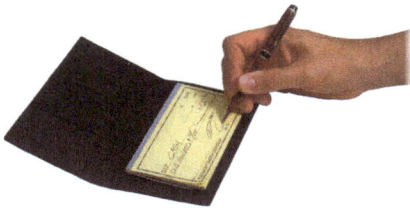 checkbook	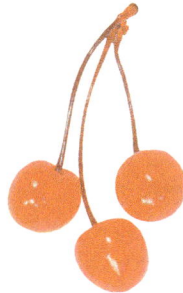 cherries	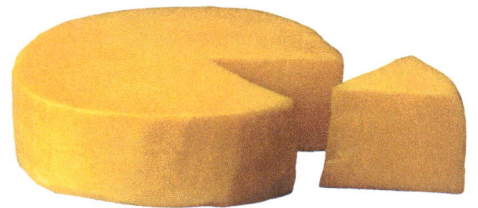 cheddar
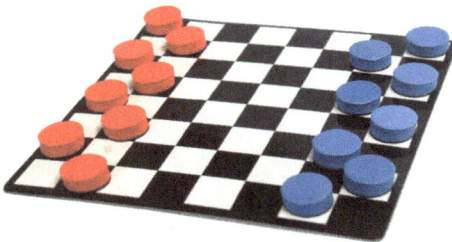 checkers	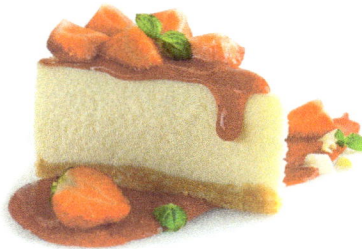 cheesecake	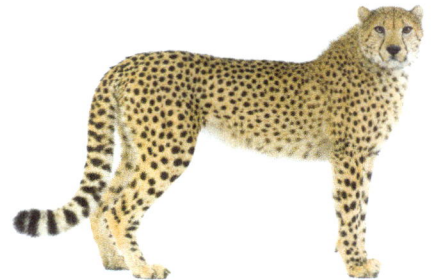 cheetah
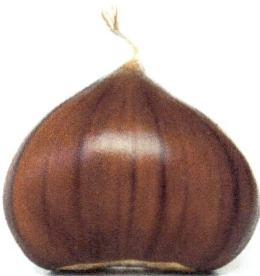 chestnut	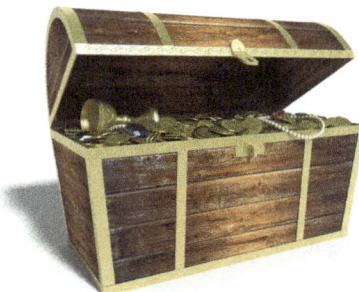 chest	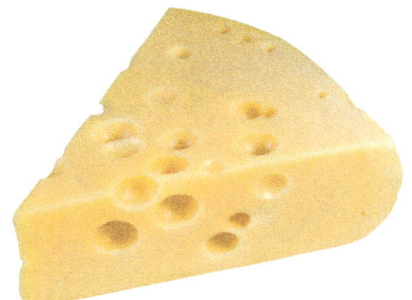 cheese

Name _____ Helper Signature _____

Speech - Language Pathologist _____ Date _____

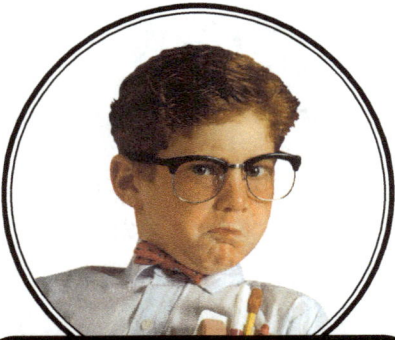

Chip

This is Chip. He chilled all the things on this page.

1. Practice your sound by saying the words on this page. (Ex. chick, chickadee, etc.). Say the last word twice.

2. Practice saying **Chip** with each of the words. (Ex. Chip chick, Chip chickadee, etc.). Say the last word pair twice.

3. Practice saying **chilled** with these words. (Ex. Chip chilled a chick, etc.). Say one of the sentences twice.

4. Practice saying **chilly** with these words. (Chip chilled the chilly chick, etc.). Say one of the expanded sentences twice.

When you finish this whole page, you will have said your sound in 100 words! Good job!

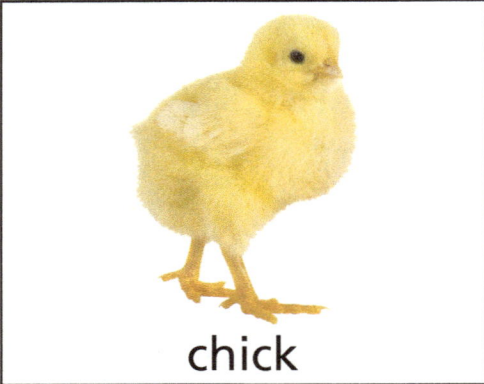	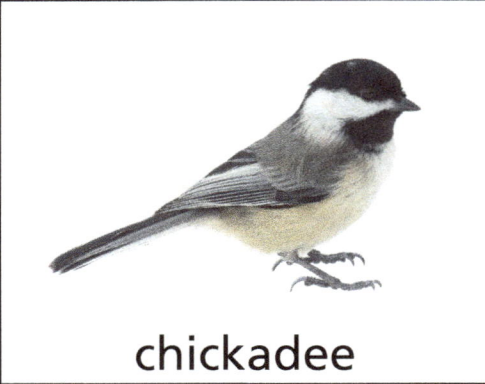	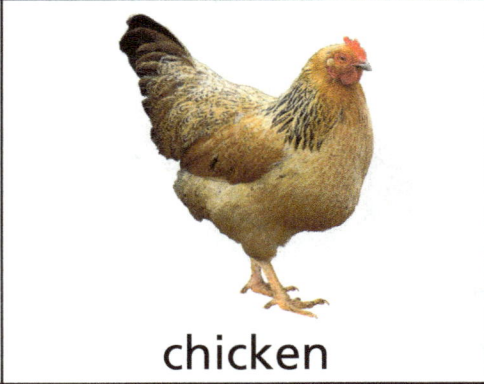
chick	chickadee	chicken
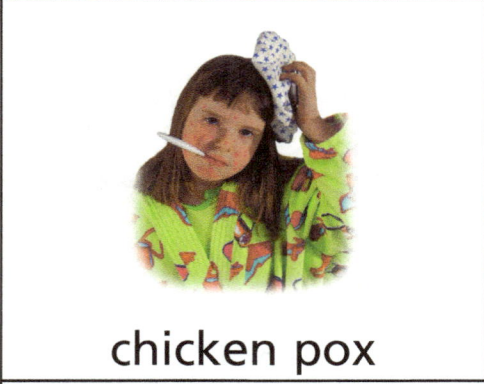	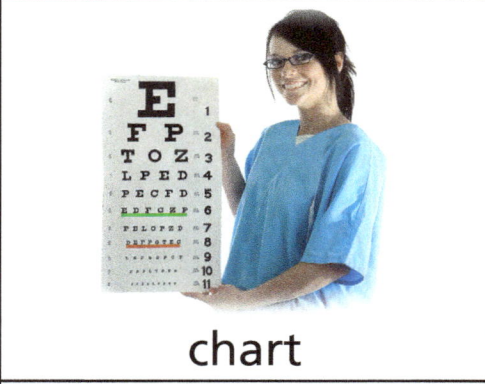	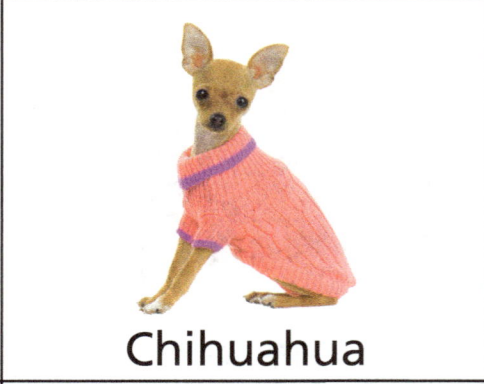
chicken pox	chart	Chihuahua
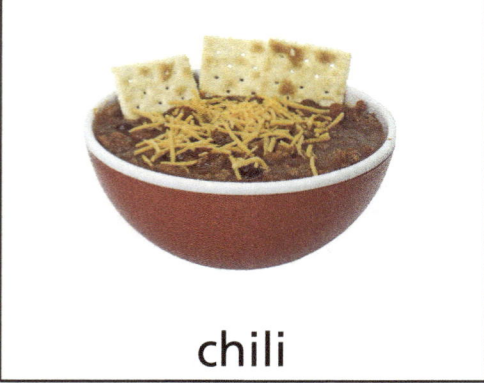	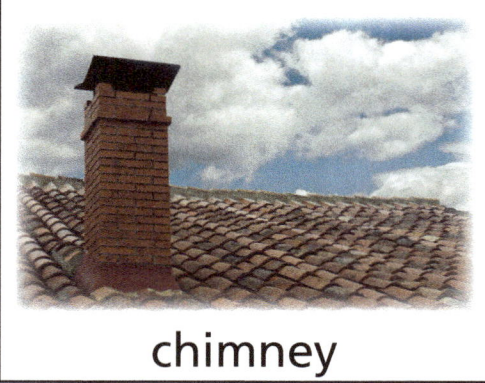	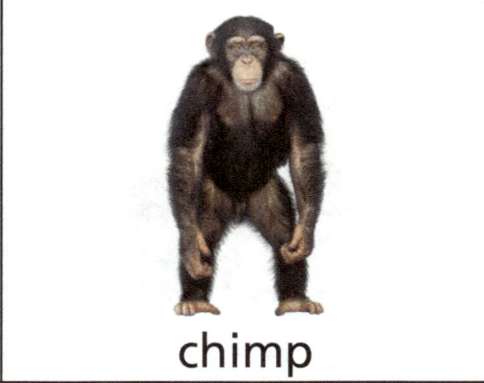
chili	chimney	chimp

Name _____

Helper Signature _____

Speech - Language Pathologist _____

Date _____

#BKCD-273 • *Say & Do® Artic Reps* • ©2015 Super Duper® Publications • www.superduperinc.com

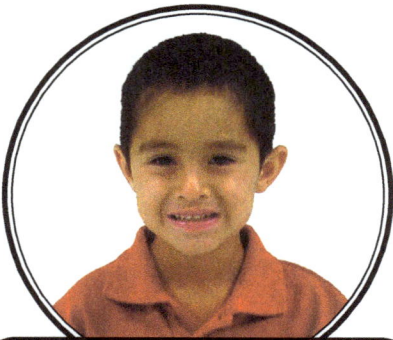

Chase

This is Chase. He chose all the things on this page.

CH – Initial Position

1. Practice your sound by saying the words on this page. (Ex. choker, choice, etc.). Say the last word twice.
2. Practice saying **Chase** with each of the words. (Ex. Chase choker, Chase choice, etc.). Say the last word pair twice.
3. Practice saying **chose** with these words. (Ex. Chase chose a choker, etc.). Say one of the sentences twice.
4. Practice saying **choosy** with these words. (Chase chose a choosy choker, etc.). Say one of the expanded sentences twice.

When you finish this whole page, you will have said your sound in 100 words! Good job!

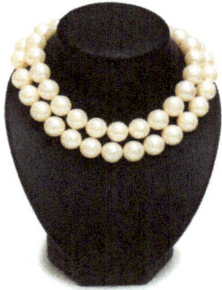

choker

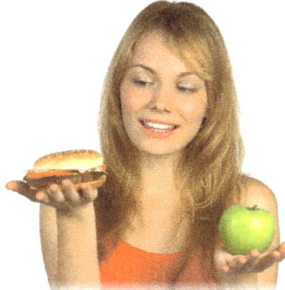

choice

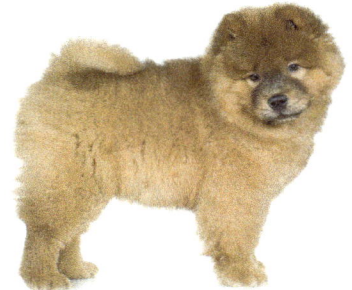

chow

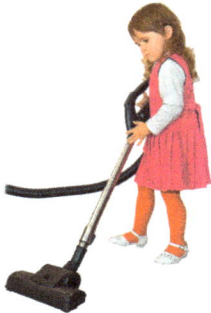

chore

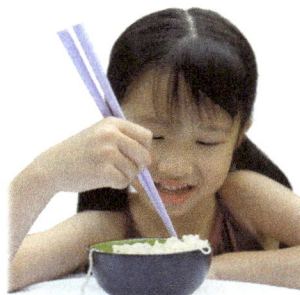

chopsticks

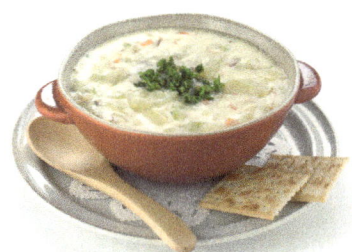

chowder

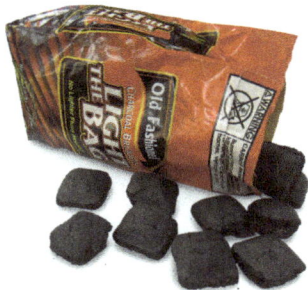

charcoal

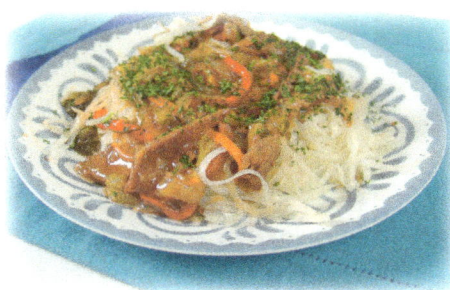

chop suey

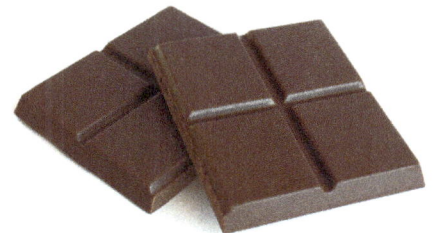

chocolate

Name _____

Helper Signature _____

Speech - Language Pathologist _____

Date _____

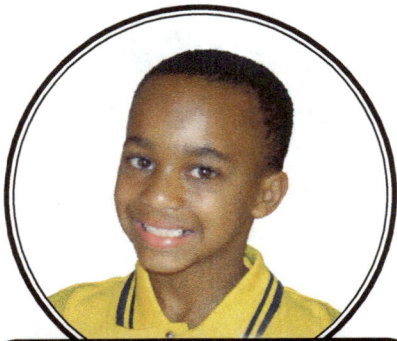

Chuck

This is Chuck. He chuckled at all the things on this page.

CH – Initial Position

1. Practice your sound by saying the words on this page. (Ex. chips, chuckles, etc.). Say the last word twice.

2. Practice saying **Chuck** with each of the words. (Ex. Chuck chips, Chuck chuckles, etc.). Say the last word pair twice.

3. Practice saying **chuckled at** with these words. (Ex. Chuck chuckled at the chips, etc.). Say one of the sentences twice.

4. Practice saying **chummy** with these words. (Chuck chuckled at the chummy chips, etc.). Say one of the expanded sentences twice.

When you finish this whole page, you will have said your sound in 100 words! Good job!

chips	chuckles	chuck wagon
chum	chunk	chess
chair	chimney	chalk

Name _____

Helper Signature _____

Speech - Language Pathologist _____

Date _____

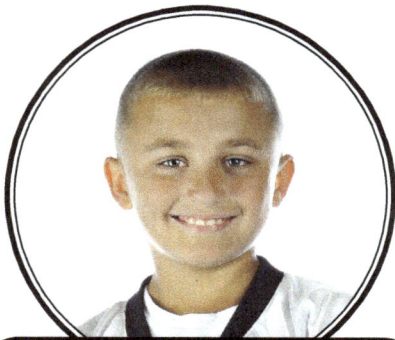

Archie

This is Archie. He watched all the things on this page.

CH – Medial Position

1. Practice your sound by saying the words on this page. (Ex. adventure, purchase, etc.). Say the last word twice.
2. Practice saying **Archie** with each of the words. (Ex. Archie adventure, Archie purchase, etc.). Say the last word pair twice.
3. Practice saying **watches** with these words. (Ex. Archie watches an adventure, etc.). Say one of the sentences twice.
4. Practice saying **miniature** with these words. (Archie watches a miniature adventure, etc.). Say one of the expanded sentences twice.

When you finish this whole page, you will have said your sound in 100 words! Good job!

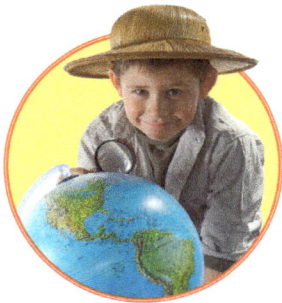 adventure	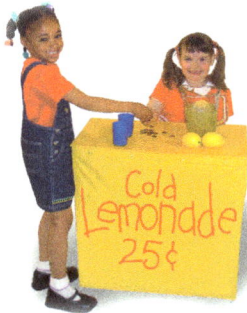 purchase	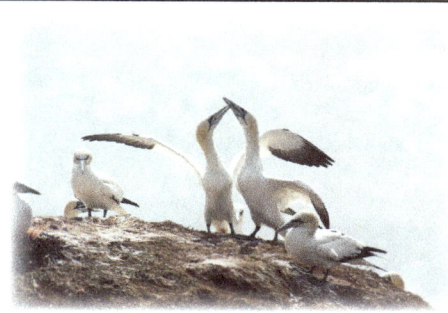 hatchery
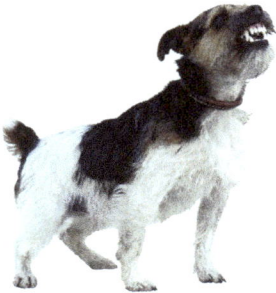 watchdog	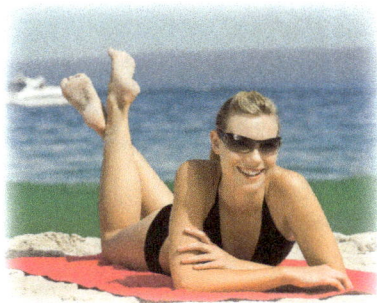 beach front	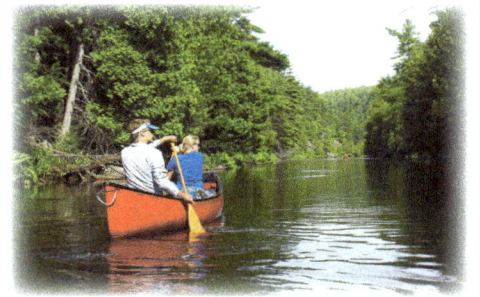 nature
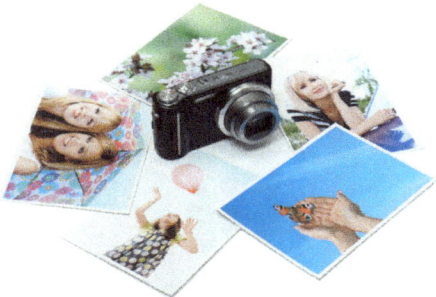 pictures	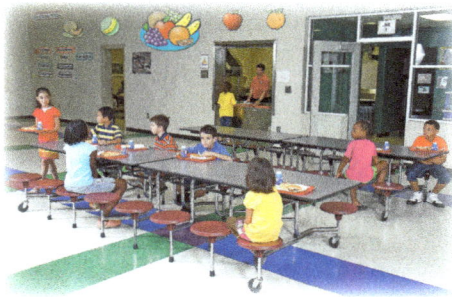 lunchroom	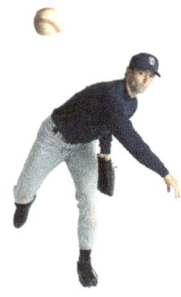 pitcher

Name _____

Helper Signature _____

Speech - Language Pathologist _____

Date _____

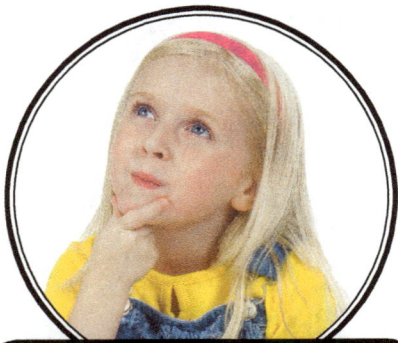

Gretchen

This is Gretchen. She pinched all the things on this page.

CH – Medial Position

1. Practice your sound by saying the words on this page. (Ex. teacher, pitcher, etc.). Say the last word twice.

2. Practice saying **Gretchen** with each of the words. (Ex. Gretchen teacher, Gretchen pitcher, etc.). Say the last word pair twice.

3. Practice saying **captures** with these words. (Ex. Gretchen captures a teacher, etc.). Say one of the sentences twice.

4. Practice saying **grouchy** with these words. (Gretchen captures the grouchy teacher, etc.). Say one of the expanded sentences twice.

When you finish this whole page, you will have said your sound in 100 words! Good job!

teacher	pitcher	poncho
witches	creature	beach bum
butcher	woodchuck	statue

Name

Helper Signature

Speech - Language Pathologist

Date

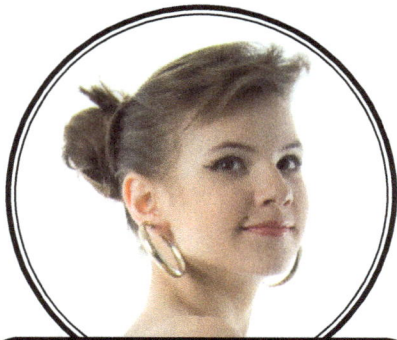

Rachel

This is Rachel. She searches for all the things on this page.

CH – Medial Position

1. Practice your sound by saying the words on this page. (Ex. benches, question, etc.). Say the last word twice.

2. Practice saying **Rachel** with each of the words. (Ex. Rachel benches, Rachel question mark, etc.). Say the last word pair twice.

3. Practice saying **searches for** with these words. (Ex. Rachel searches for benches, etc.). Say one of the sentences twice.

4. Practice saying **future** with these words. (Rachel searches for future benches, etc.). Say one of the expanded sentences twice.

When you finish this whole page, you will have said your sound in 100 words! Good job!

benches	question mark	kitchen
pasture	orchard	stretcher
wheelchair	branches	riches

Name _____

Helper Signature _____

Speech - Language Pathologist _____

Date _____

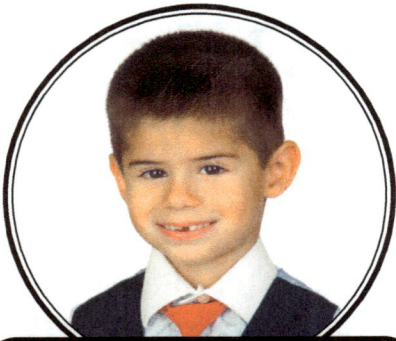

Mitchell

This is Mitchell. He touches all the things on this page.

1. Practice your sound by saying the words on this page. (Ex. anchovies, beach ball, etc.). Say the last word twice.

2. Practice saying **Mitchell** with each of the words. (Ex. Mitchell anchovies, Mitchell beach ball, etc.). Say the last word pair twice.

3. Practice saying **touches** with these words. (Ex. Mitchell touches anchovies, etc.). Say one of the sentences twice.

4. Practice saying **crunchy** with these words. (Mitchell touches crunchy anchovies, etc.). Say one of the expanded sentences twice.

When you finish this whole page, you will have said your sound in 100 words! Good job!

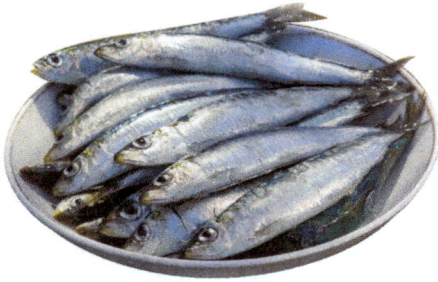	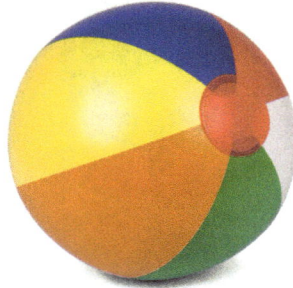	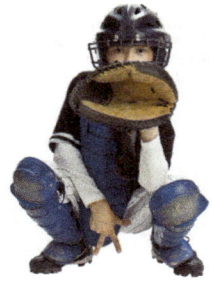
anchovies	beach ball	catcher
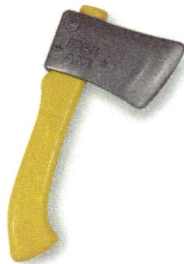	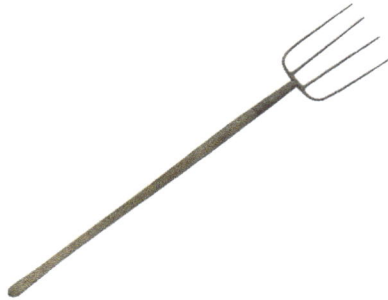	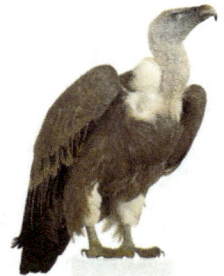
hatchet	pitchfork	vulture
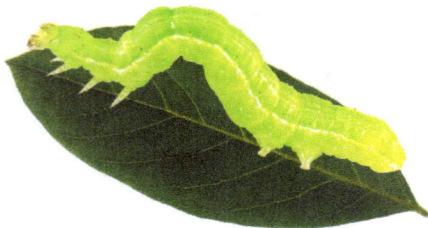	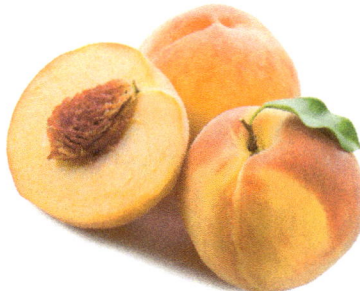	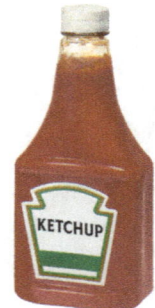
inchworm	peaches	ketchup

Name _____

Helper Signature _____

Speech - Language Pathologist _____

Date _____

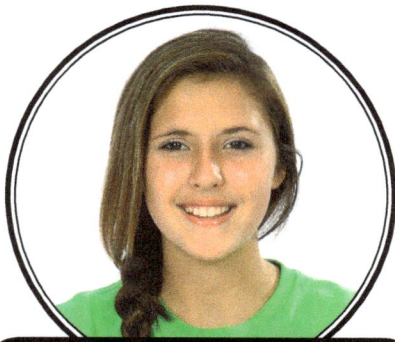

Blanche

This is Blanche. She will sketch all the things on this page.

1. Practice your sound by saying the words on this page. (Ex. watch, avalanche, etc.). Say the last word twice.

2. Practice saying **Blanche** with each of the words. (Ex. Blanche watch, Blanche avalanche, etc.). Say the last word pair twice.

3. Practice saying **will sketch** with these words. (Ex. Blanche will sketch a watch, etc.). Say one of the sentences twice.

4. Practice saying **each** with these words. (Blanche will sketch each watch, etc.). Say one of the expanded sentences twice.

   When you finish this whole page, you will have said your sound in 100 words! Good job!

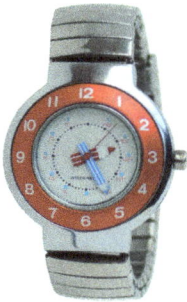 watch	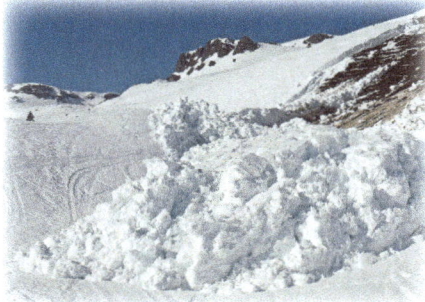 avalanche	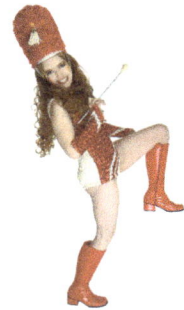 march
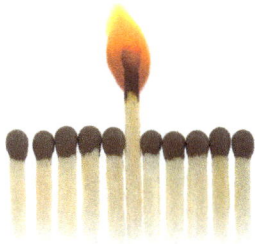 match	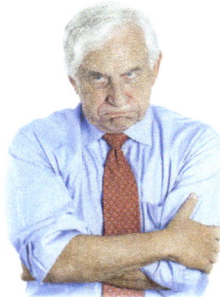 grouch	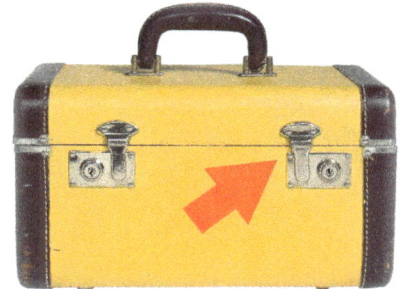 latch
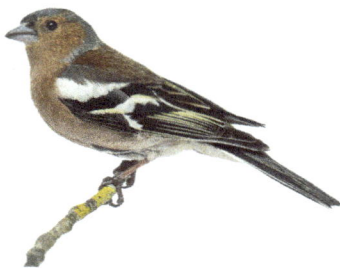 finch	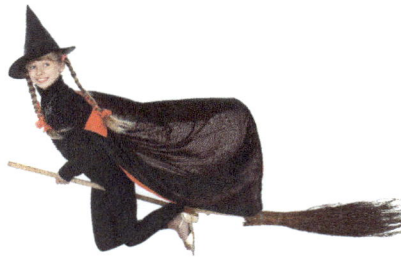 witch	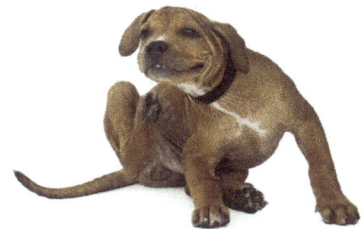 scratch

Name _____

Helper Signature _____

Speech - Language Pathologist _____

Date _____

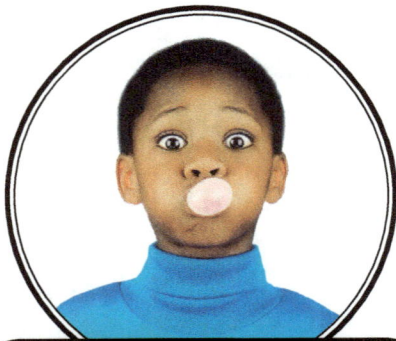

Fletch

This is Fletch. He can reach all the things on this page.

CH – Final Position

1. Practice your sound by saying the words on this page. (Ex. porch, beach, etc.). Say the last word twice.

2. Practice saying **Fletch** with each of the words. (Ex. Fletch porch, Fletch beach, etc.). Say the last word pair twice.

3. Practice saying **can reach** with these words. (Ex. Fletch can reach the porch, etc.). Say one of the sentences twice.

4. Practice saying **Dutch** with these words. (Fletch can reach the Dutch porch, etc.). Say one of the expanded sentences twice.

When you finish this whole page, you will have said your sound in 100 words! Good job!

porch	beach	bench
wrench	ranch	patch
briar patch	bleach	perch

Name _____

Speech - Language Pathologist _____

Helper Signature _____

Date _____

#BKCD-273 • *Say & Do® Artic Reps* • ©2015 Super Duper® Publications • www.superduperinc.com

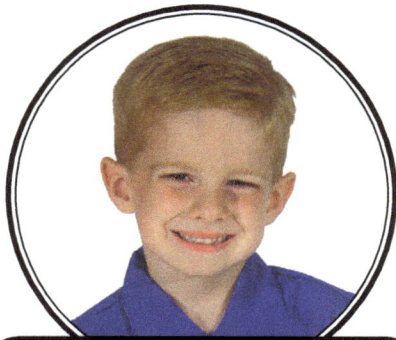

Mitch

This is Mitch. He can teach all the things on this page.

1. Practice your sound by saying the words on this page. (Ex. coach, stitch, etc.). Say the last word twice.

2. Practice saying **Mitch** with each of the words. (Ex. Mitch coach, Mitch stitch, etc.). Say the last word pair twice.

3. Practice saying **can teach** with these words. (Ex. Mitch can teach the coach, etc.). Say one of the sentences twice.

4. Practice saying **French** with these words. (Mitch can teach the French coach, etc.). Say one of the expanded sentences twice.

When you finish this whole page, you will have said your sound in 100 words! Good job!

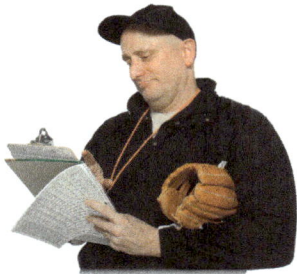 coach	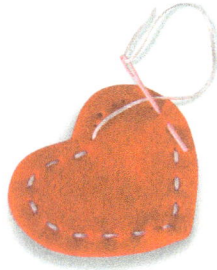 stitch	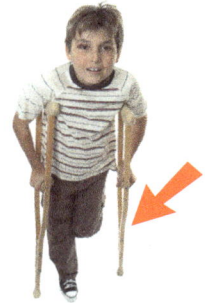 crutch
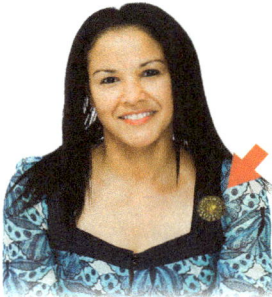 brooch	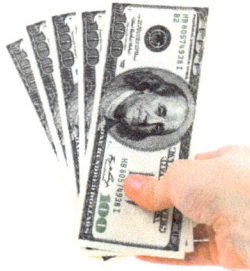 rich	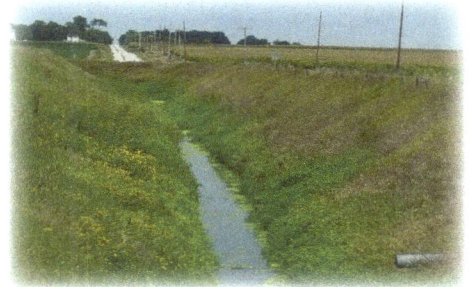 ditch
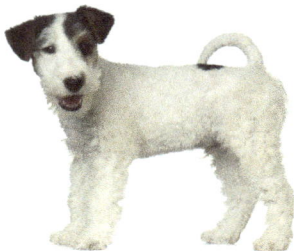 pooch	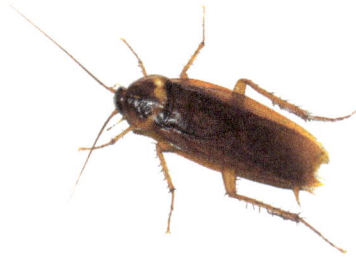 roach	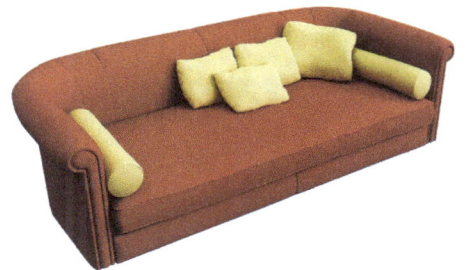 couch

Name _____

Helper Signature _____

Speech - Language Pathologist _____

Date _____

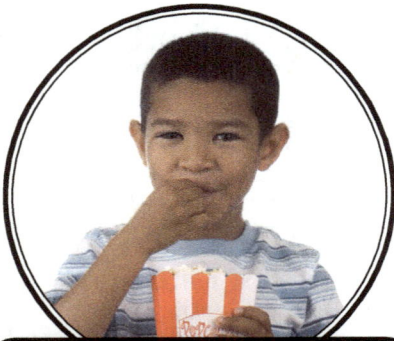

Butch

This is Butch. He can munch all the things on this page.

CH – Final Position

1. Practice your sound by saying the words on this page. (Ex. peach, ostrich, etc.). Say the last word twice.

2. Practice saying **Butch** with each of the words. (Ex. Butch peach, Butch ostrich, etc.). Say the last word pair twice.

3. Practice saying **can munch** with these words. (Ex. Butch can munch a peach, etc.). Say one of the sentences twice.

4. Practice saying **rich** with these words. (Butch can munch a rich peach, etc.). Say one of the expanded sentences twice.

When you finish this whole page, you will have said your sound in 100 words! Good job!

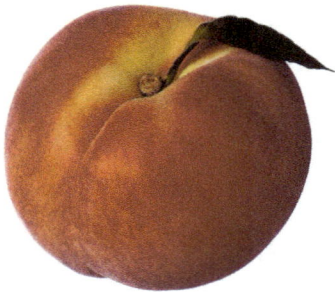

peach

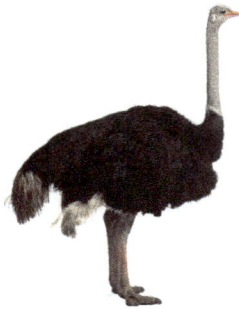

ostrich

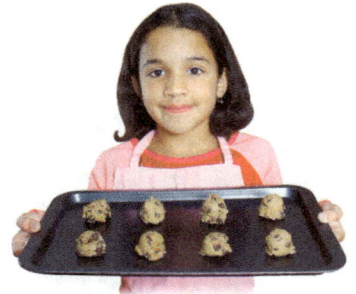

batch

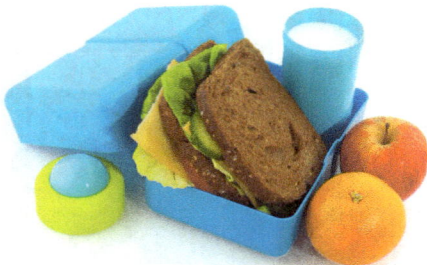

lunch

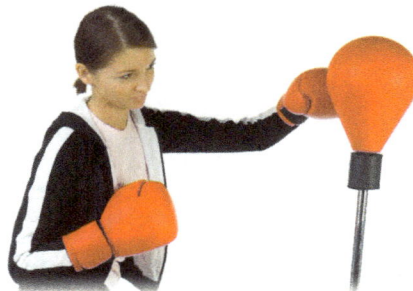

punch

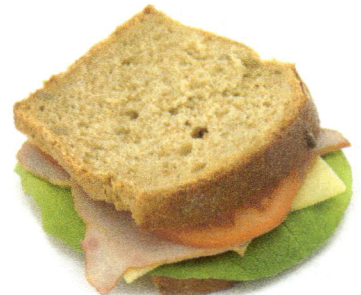

sandwich

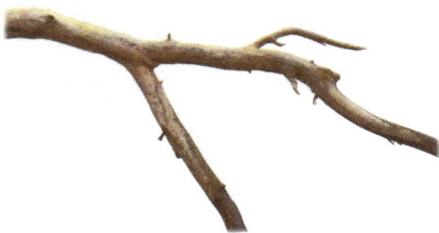

branch

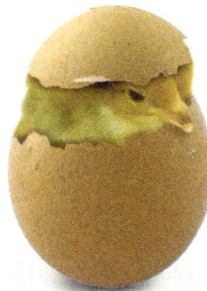

hatch

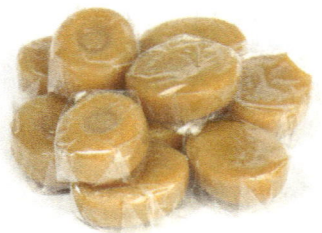

butterscotch

Name _____

Helper Signature _____

Speech - Language Pathologist _____

Date _____

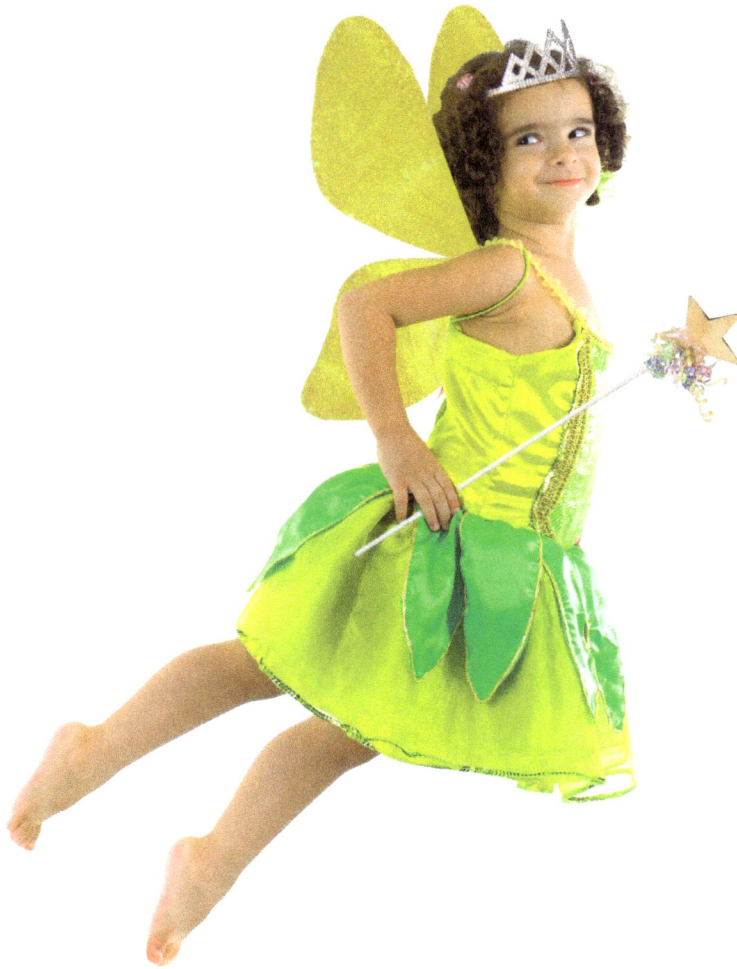

F

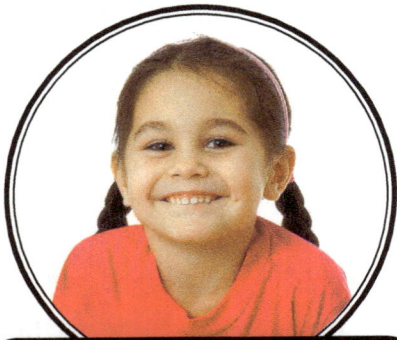

Fay

This is Fay. She faced all the things on this page.

F – Initial Position

1. Practice your sound by saying the words on this page. (Ex. fan, falcon, etc.). Say the last word twice.

2. Practice saying **Fay** with each of the words. (Ex. Fay fan, Fay falcon, etc.). Say the last word pair twice.

3. Practice saying **faced** with these words. (Ex. Fay faced a fan, etc.). Say one of the sentences twice.

4. Practice saying **famous** with these words. (Fay faced a famous fan, etc.). Say one of the expanded sentences twice.

When you have finished this whole page you will have said your sound in 100 words! Good job!

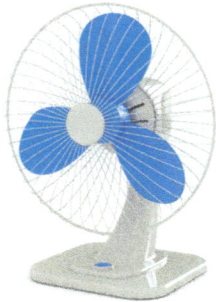 fan	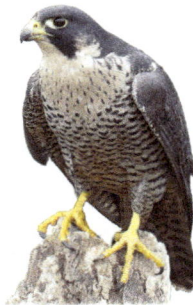 falcon	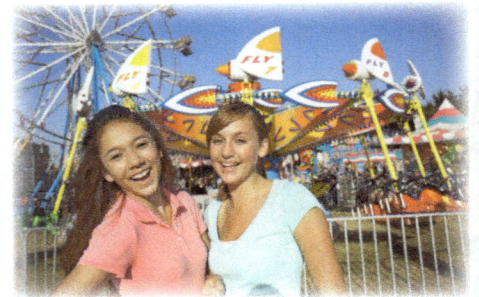 fair
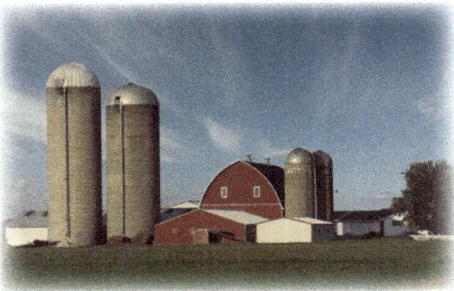 farm	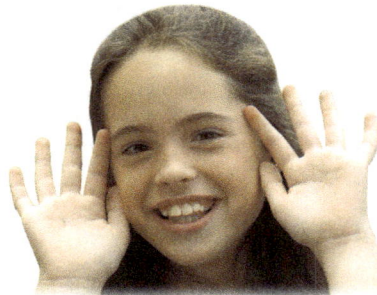 face	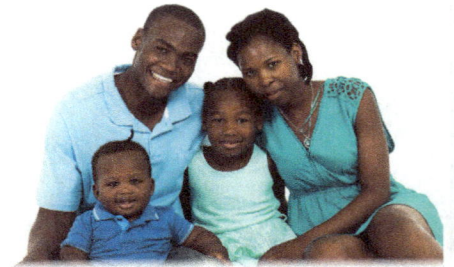 family
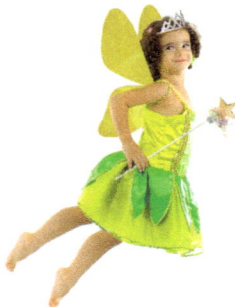 fairy	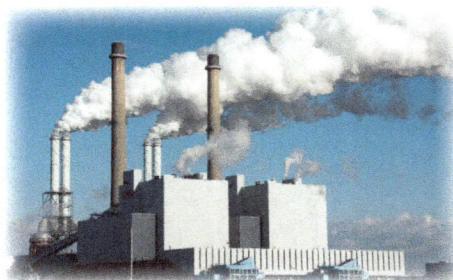 factory	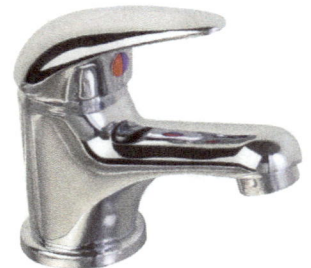 faucet

Name _____

Helper Signature _____

Speech - Language Pathologist _____

Date _____

#BKCD-273 • *Say & Do® Artic Reps* • ©2015 Super Duper® Publications • www.superduperinc.com

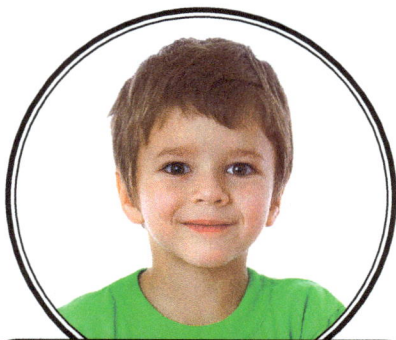

Felix

This is Felix. He fed all the things on this page.

1. Practice your sound by saying the words on this page. (Ex. feathers, ferns, etc.). Say the last word twice.
2. Practice saying **Felix** with each of the words. (Ex. Felix feathers, Felix ferns, etc.). Say the last word pair twice.
3. Practice saying **fed** with these words. (Ex. Felix fed feathers, etc.). Say one of the sentences twice.
4. Practice saying **a few** with these words. (Felix fed a few feathers, etc.). Say one of the expanded sentences twice.

When you have finished this whole page you will have said your sound in 100 words! Good job!

feathers	ferns	feet
females	ferrets	fields
funnels	fences	Ferris wheels

Name _____

Helper Signature _____

Speech - Language Pathologist _____

Date _____

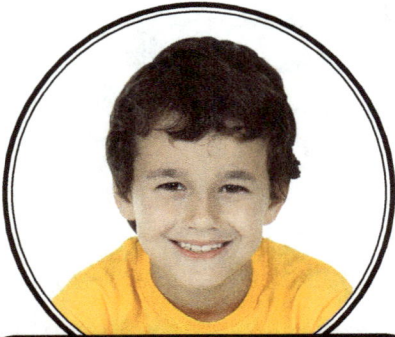

Phil

This is Phil. He fixed all the things on this page.

F – Initial Position

1. Practice your sound by saying the words on this page. (Ex. fire trucks, files, etc.). Say the last word twice.

2. Practice saying **Phil** with each of the words. (Ex. Phil fire trucks, Phil files, etc.). Say the last word pair twice.

3. Practice saying **fixed** with these words. (Ex. Phil fixed fire trucks, etc.). Say one of the sentences twice.

4. Practice saying **five** with these words. (Phil fixed five fire trucks, etc.). Say one of the expanded sentences twice.

When you have finished this whole page you will have said your sound in 100 words! Good job!

fire trucks	files	films
fingers	fires	fish
fire escapes	fishbowls	filters

Name _____

Speech - Language Pathologist _____

Helper Signature _____

Date _____

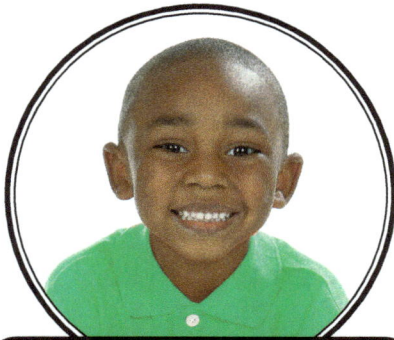

Fonzie

This is Fonzie. He found all the things on this page.

F – Initial Position

1. Practice your sound by saying the words on this page. (Ex. fountains, foxes, etc.). Say the last word twice.

2. Practice saying **Fonzie** with each of the words. (Ex. Fonzie fountains, Fonzie foxes, etc.). Say the last word pair twice.

3. Practice saying **found** with these words. (Ex. Fonzie found fountains, etc.). Say one of the sentences twice.

4. Practice saying **four** with these words. (Fonzie found four fountains, etc.). Say one of the expanded sentences twice.

When you have finished this whole page you will have said your sound in 100 words! Good job!

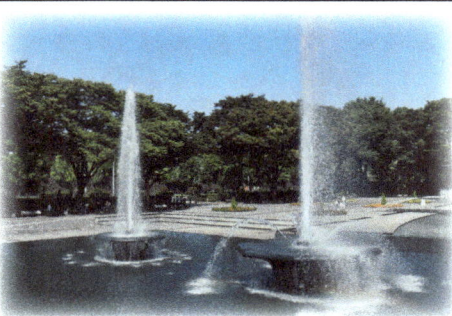 fountains	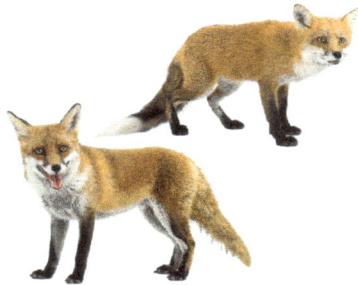 foxes	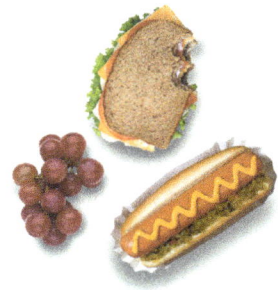 foods
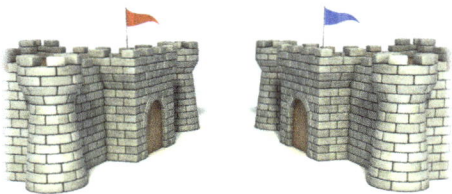 forts	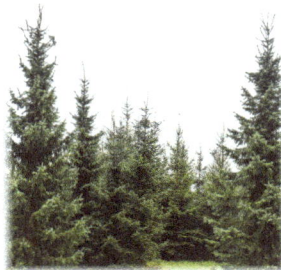 forests	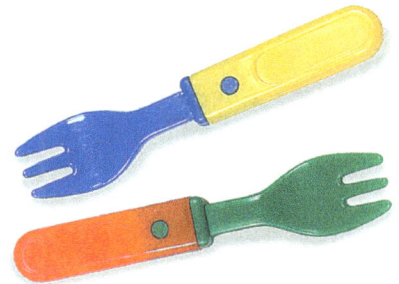 forks
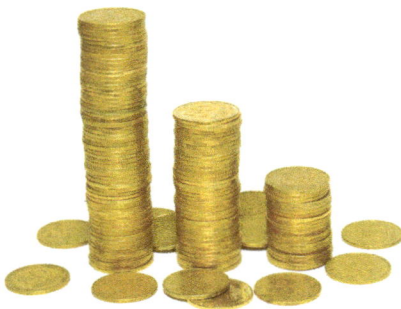 fortunes	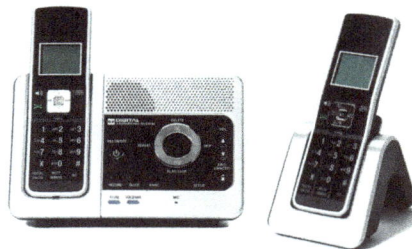 phones	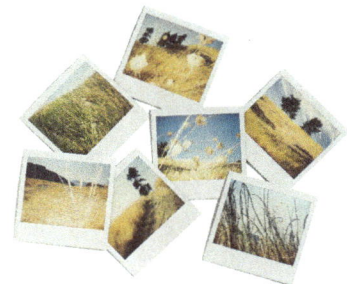 photos

Name _____

Helper Signature _____

Speech - Language Pathologist _____

Date _____

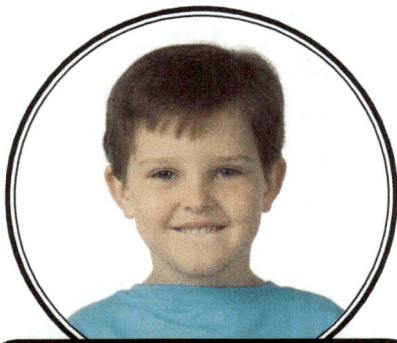

Fulton

This is Fulton. He fussed about all the things on this page.

1. Practice your sound by saying the words on this page. (Ex. fudge, fever, etc.). Say the last word twice.

2. Practice saying **Fulton** with each of the words. (Ex. Fulton fudge, Fulton fever, etc.). Say the last word pair twice.

3. Practice saying **fussed about** with these words. (Ex. Fulton fussed about fudge, etc.). Say one of the sentences twice.

4. Practice saying **funny** with these words. (Fulton fussed about the funny fudge, etc.). Say one of the expanded sentences twice.

When you have finished this whole page you will have said your sound in 100 words! Good job!

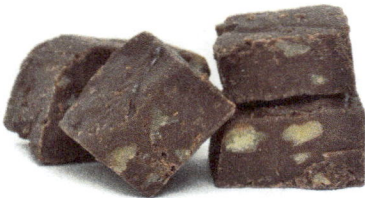 fudge	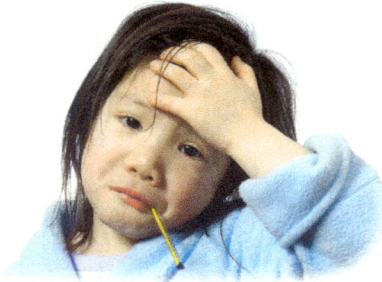 fever	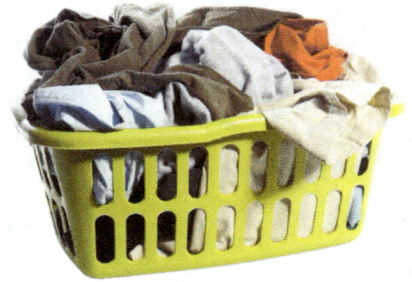 full basket
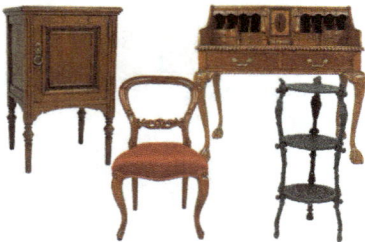 furniture	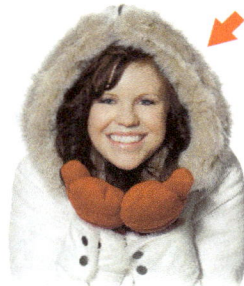 fur	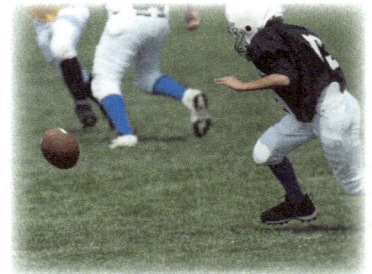 fumble
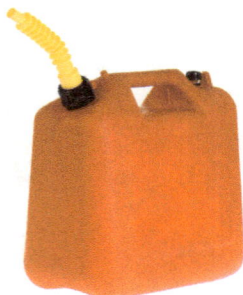 fuel	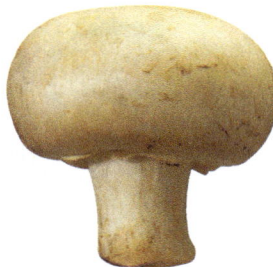 fungus	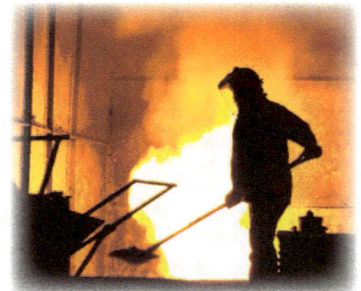 furnace

Name _____

Helper Signature _____

Speech - Language Pathologist

Date _____

#BKCD-273 • *Say & Do*® Artic Reps • ©2015 Super Duper® Publications • www.superduperinc.com

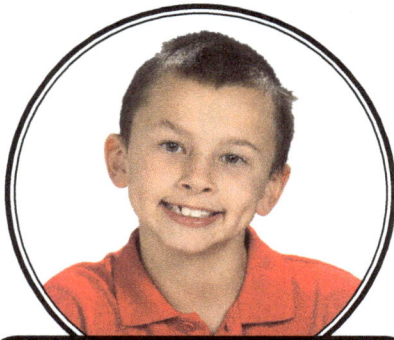

Alphie

This is Alphie. He confessed to all the things on this page.

1. Practice your sound by saying the words on this page. (Ex. crayfish, lifeguard, etc.). Say the last word twice.

2. Practice saying **Alphie** with each of the words. (Ex. Alphie crayfish, Alphie lifeguard, etc.). Say the last word pair twice.

3. Practice saying **confessed to** with these words. (Ex. Alphie confessed to the crayfish, etc.). Say one of the sentences twice.

4. Practice saying **awful** with these words. (Alphie confessed to the awful crayfish, etc.). Say one of the expanded sentences twice.

When you have finished this whole page you will have said your sound in 100 words! Good job!

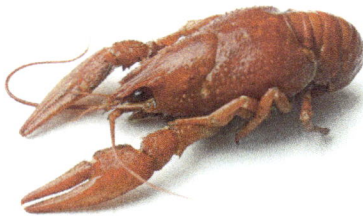

crayfish

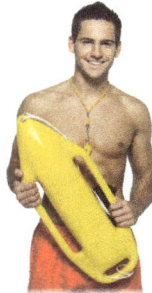

lifeguard

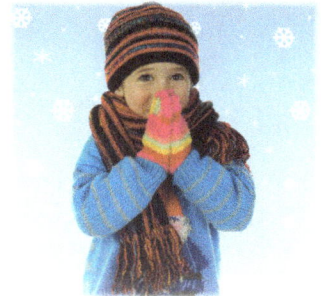

snowfall

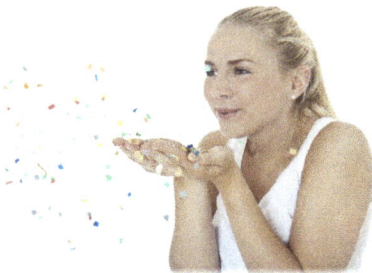

confetti

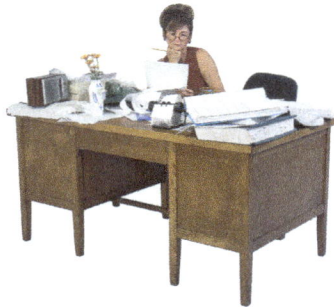

office

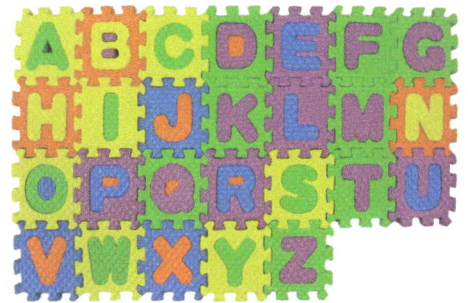

alphabet

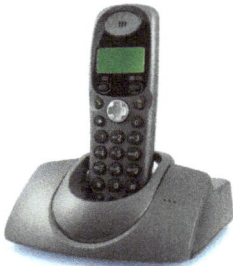

telephone

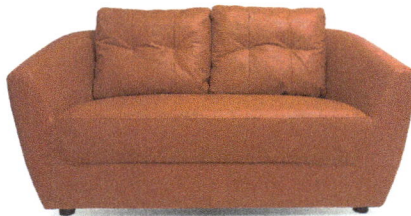

sofa

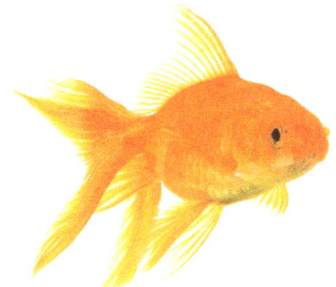

goldfish

Name _____

Helper Signature _____

Speech - Language Pathologist _____

Date _____

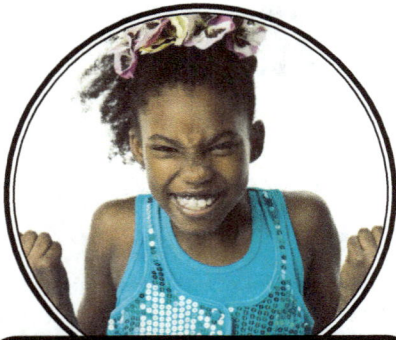

Tiffany

This is Tiffany. She defended all the things on this page.

1. Practice your sound by saying the words on this page. (Ex. infant, muffin, etc.). Say the last word twice.

2. Practice saying **Tiffany** with each of the words. (Ex. Tiffany infant, Tiffany muffin, etc.). Say the last word pair twice.

3. Practice saying **defended** with these words. (Ex. Tiffany defended the infant, etc.). Say one of the sentences twice.

4. Practice saying **chiffon** with these words. (Tiffany defended a chiffon infant, etc.). Say one of the expanded sentences twice.

When you have finished this whole page you will have said your sound in 100 words! Good job!

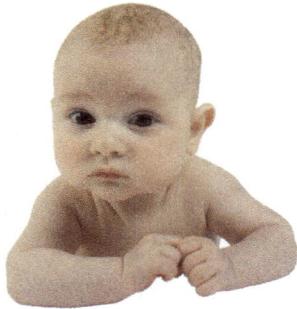 infant	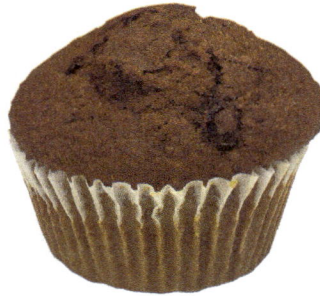 muffin	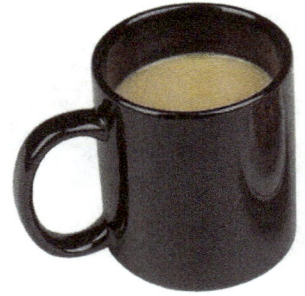 coffee
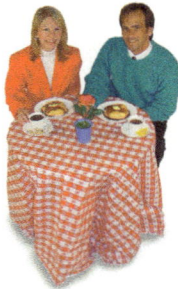 cafe	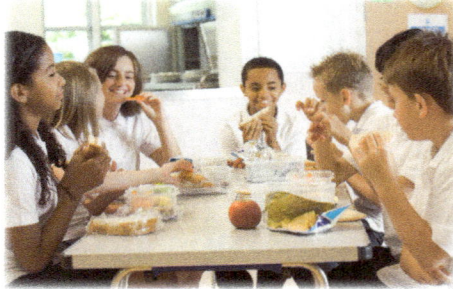 cafeteria	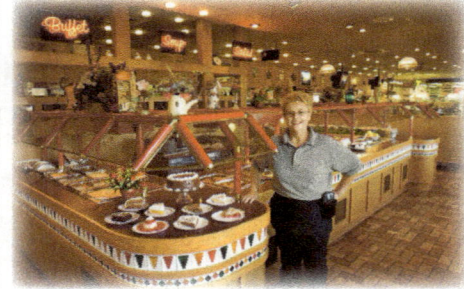 buffet
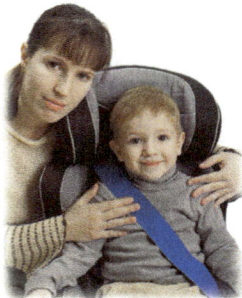 safety belt	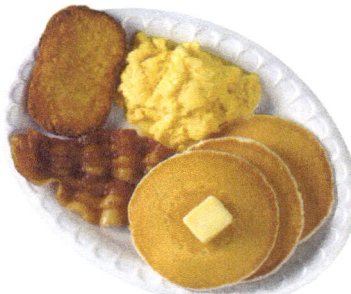 breakfast	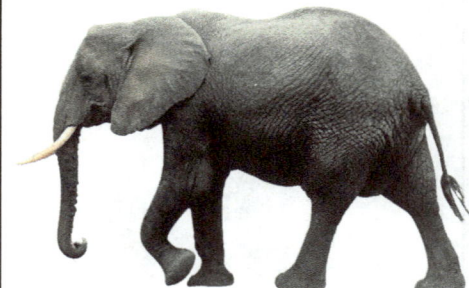 elephant

Name _____

Speech - Language Pathologist _____

Helper Signature _____

Date _____

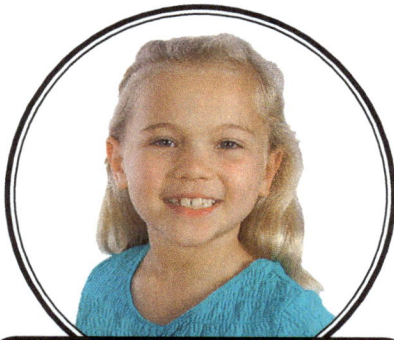

Sophie

This is Sophie. She prefers all the things on this page.

F – Medial Position

1. Practice your sound by saying the words on this page. (Ex. lifeboat, trophy, etc.). Say the last word twice.

2. Practice saying **Sophie** with each of the words. (Ex. Sophie lifeboat, Sophie trophy, etc.). Say the last word pair twice.

3. Practice saying **prefers** with these words. (Ex. Sophie prefers a lifeboat, etc.). Say one of the sentences twice.

4. Practice saying **low-fat** with these words. (Sophie prefers the low-fat lifeboat, etc.). Say one of the expanded sentences twice.

When you have finished this whole page you will have said your sound in 100 words! Good job!

lifeboat	trophy	headphones
saxophone	rainfall	alphabet soup
microphone	taffy	buffalo

Name _____

Helper Signature _____

Speech - Language Pathologist _____

Date _____

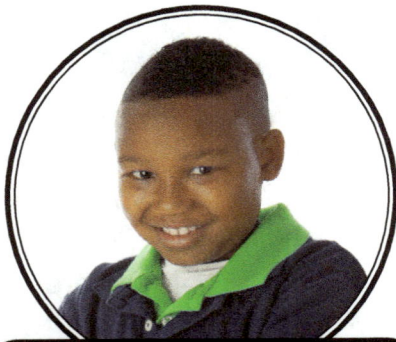

Clifford

This is Clifford. He refunded all the things on this page.

1. Practice your sound by saying the words on this page. (Ex. gopher, amphibian, etc.). Say the last word twice.
2. Practice saying **Clifford** with each of the words. (Ex. Clifford gopher, Clifford amphibian, etc.). Say the last word pair twice.
3. Practice saying **refunded** with these words. (Ex. Clifford refunded the gopher, etc.). Say one of the sentences twice.
4. Practice saying **playful** with these words. (Clifford refunded a playful gopher, etc.). Say one of the expanded sentences twice.

When you have finished this whole page you will have said your sound in 100 words! Good job!

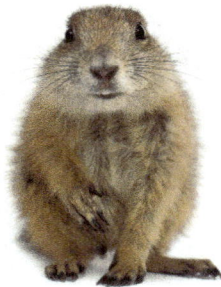 gopher	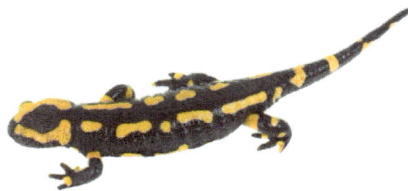 amphibian	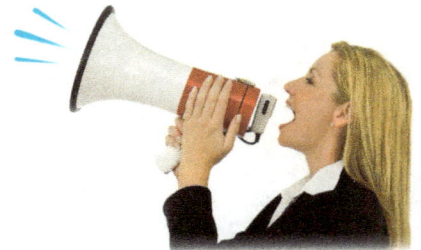 megaphone
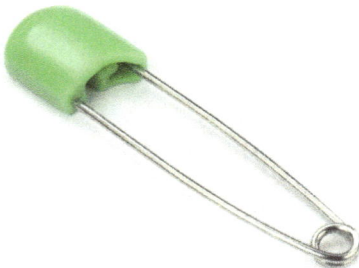 safety pin	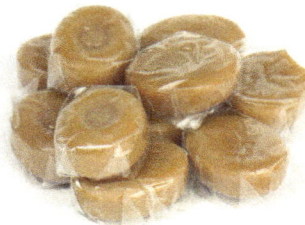 toffee	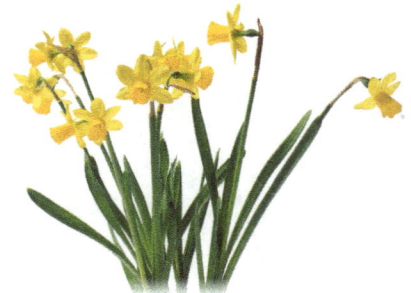 daffodil
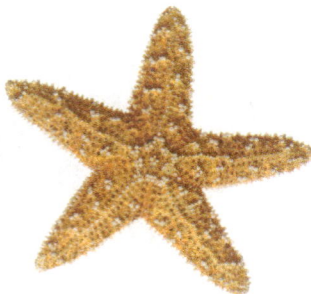 starfish	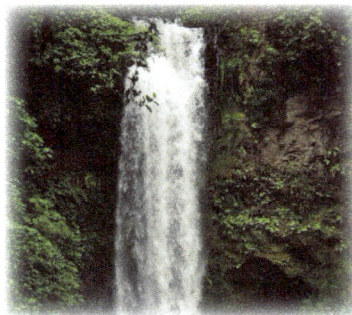 waterfall	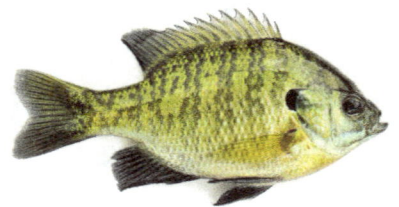 sunfish

Name _____

Helper Signature _____

Speech - Language Pathologist _____

Date _____

#BKCD-273 • *Say & Do® Artic Reps* • ©2015 Super Duper® Publications • www.superduperinc.com

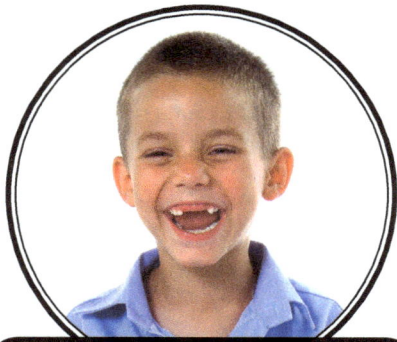

Ralph

This is Ralph. He can laugh at all the things on this page.

1. Practice your sound by saying the words on this page. (Ex. calf, wife, etc.). Say the last word twice.

2. Practice saying **Ralph** with each of the words. (Ex. Ralph calf, Ralph wife, etc.). Say the last word pair twice.

3. Practice saying **can laugh** at with these words. (Ex. Ralph can laugh at a calf, etc.). Say one of the sentences twice.

4. Practice saying **rough** with these words. (Ralph can laugh at a rough calf, etc.). Say one of the expanded sentences twice.

When you have finished this whole page you will have said your sound in 100 words! Good job!

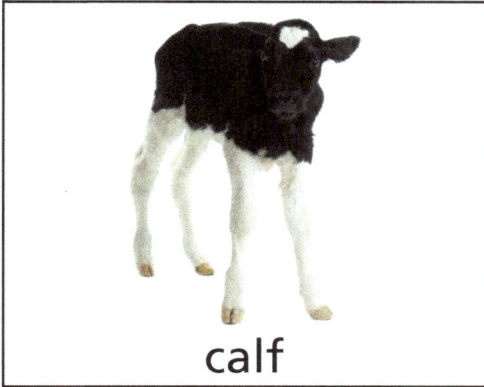

calf

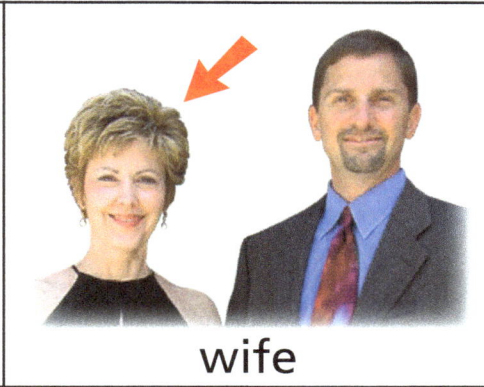

wife

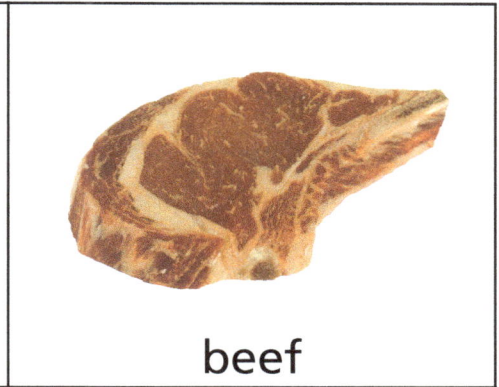

beef

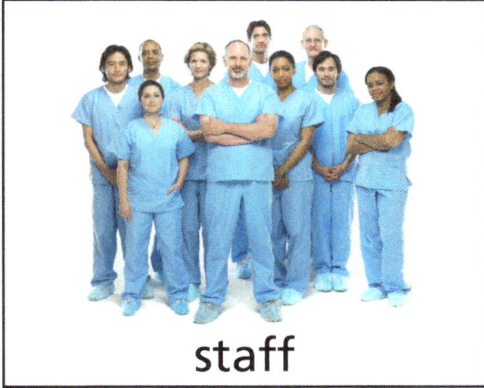

staff

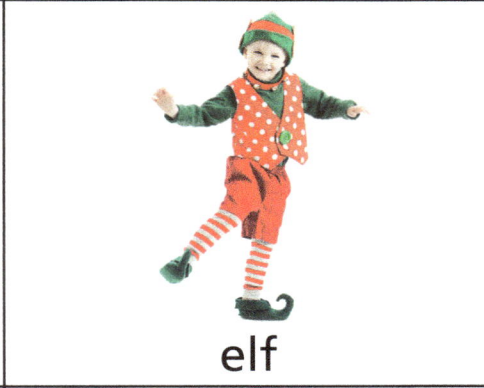

elf

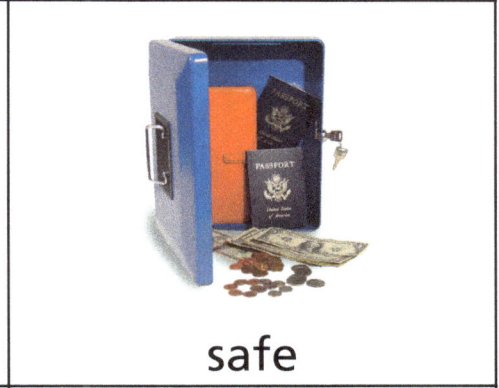

safe

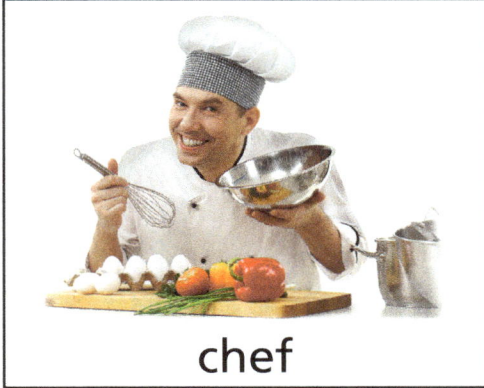

chef

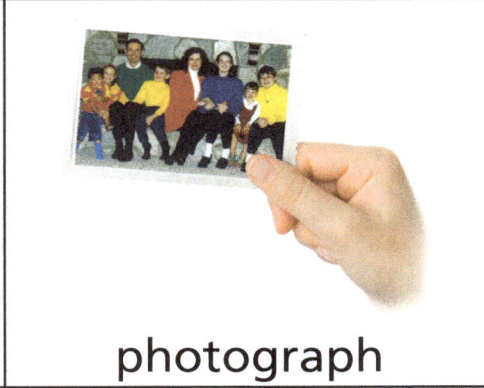

photograph

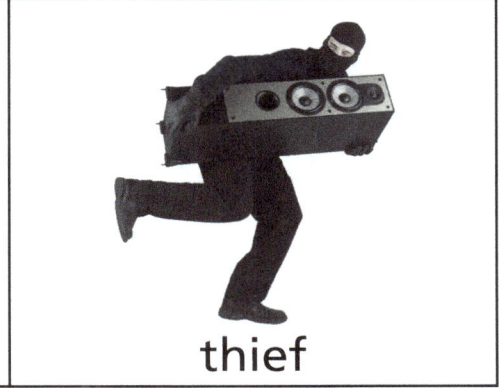

thief

Name _____

Helper Signature _____

Speech - Language Pathologist _____

Date _____

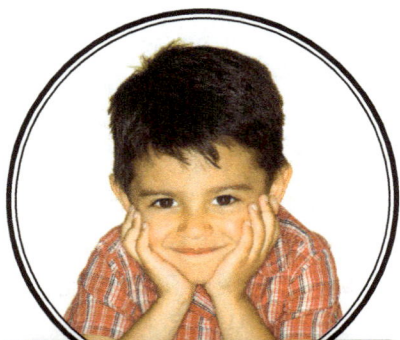

Jeff

This is Jeff. He takes off all the things on this page.

F – Final Position

1. Practice your sound by saying the words on this page. (Ex. dandruff, chief, etc.). Say the last word twice.

2. Practice saying **Jeff** with each of the words. (Ex. Jeff dandruff, Jeff chief, etc.). Say the last word pair twice.

3. Practice saying **takes off** with these words. (Ex. Jeff takes off dandruff, etc.). Say one of the sentences twice.

4. Practice saying **stiff** with these words. (Jeff takes off stiff dandruff, etc.). Say one of the expanded sentences twice.

When you have finished this whole page you will have said your sound in 100 words! Good job!

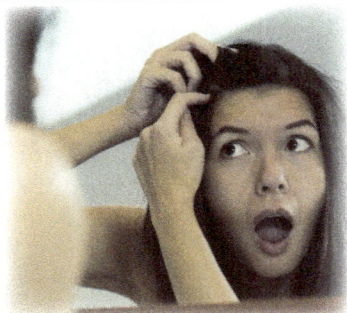 dandruff	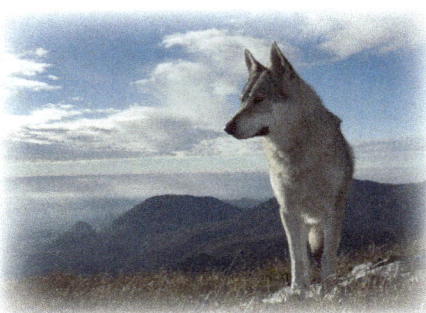 wolf	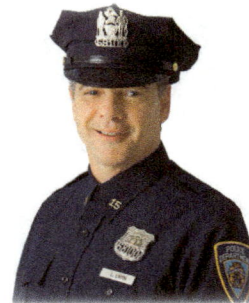 sheriff
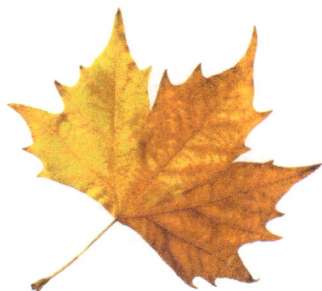 leaf	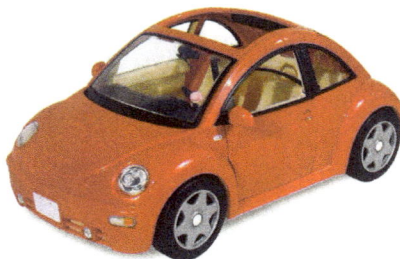 sunroof	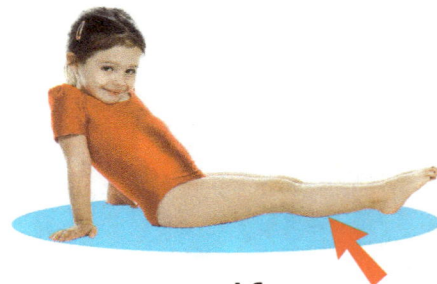 calf
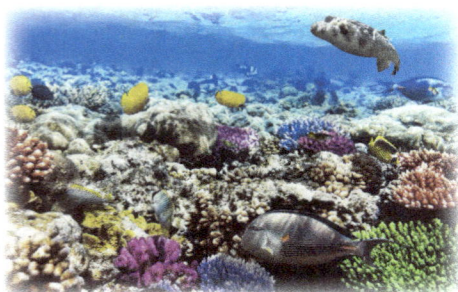 reef	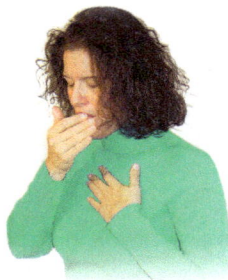 cough	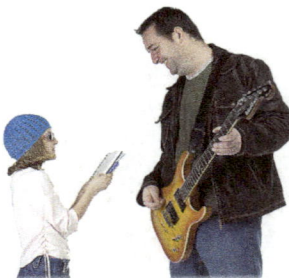 autograph

Name _____

Helper Signature _____

Speech - Language Pathologist _____

Date _____

#BKCD-273 • *Say & Do® Artic Reps* • ©2015 Super Duper® Publications • www.superduperinc.com

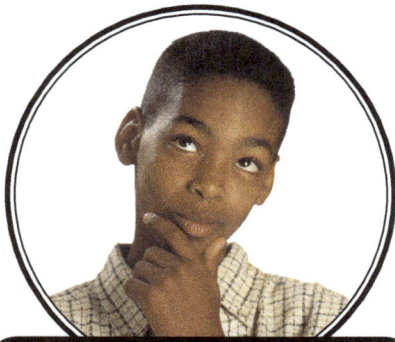

Cliff

This is Cliff. He got off all the things on this page.

F – Final Position

1. Practice your sound by saying the words on this page. (Ex. roof, cliff, etc.). Say the last word twice.

2. Practice saying **Cliff** with each of the words. (Ex. Cliff roof, Cliff cliff, etc.). Say the last word pair twice.

3. Practice saying **got off** with these words. (Ex. Cliff got off the roof, etc.). Say one of the sentences twice.

4. Practice saying **gruff** with these words. (Cliff got off a gruff roof, etc.). Say one of the expanded sentences twice.

When you have finished this whole page you will have said your sound in 100 words! Good job!

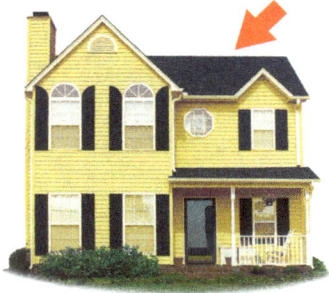

roof

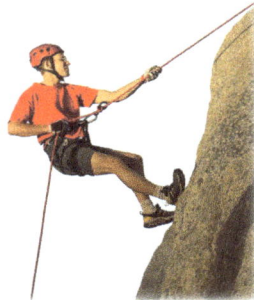

cliff

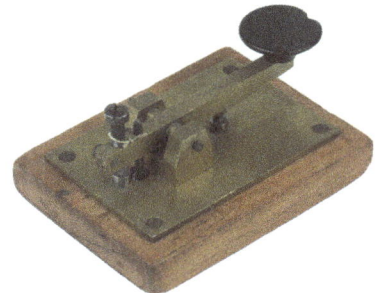

telegraph

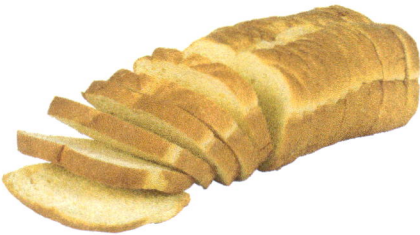

loaf

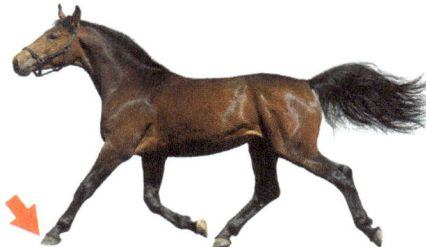

hoof

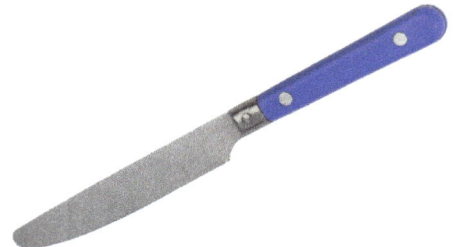

knife

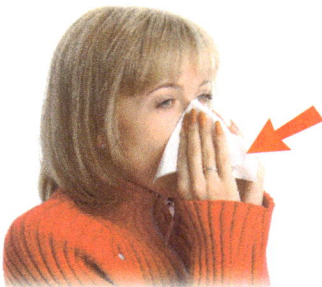

handkerchief

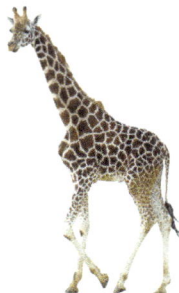

giraffe

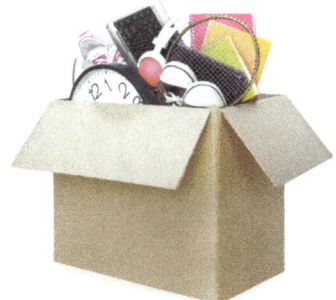

stuff

Name _____

Helper Signature _____

Speech - Language Pathologist _____

Date _____

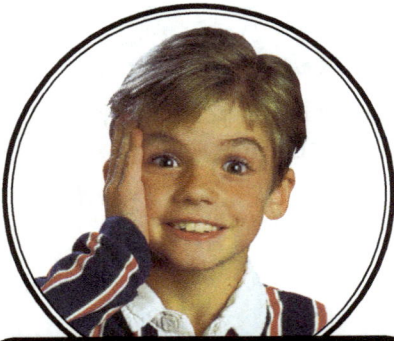

Duff

This is Duff. He cuts off all the things on this page.

F – Final Position

1. Practice your sound by saying the words on this page. (Ex. graph, cuff, etc.). Say the last word twice.

2. Practice saying **Duff** with each of the words. (Ex. Duff graph, Duff cuff, etc.). Say the last word pair twice.

3. Practice saying **cuts off** with these words. (Ex. Duff cuts off a graph, etc.). Say one of the sentences twice.

4. Practice saying **tough** with these words. (Duff cuts off a tough graph, etc.). Say one of the expanded sentences twice.

When you have finished this whole page you will have said your sound in 100 words! Good job!

graph	cuff	muff
kerchief	laugh	handcuff
half	trough	enough

Name _____

Helper Signature _____

Speech - Language Pathologist _____

Date _____

#BKCD-273 • *Say & Do® Artic Reps* • ©2015 Super Duper® Publications • www.superduperinc.com

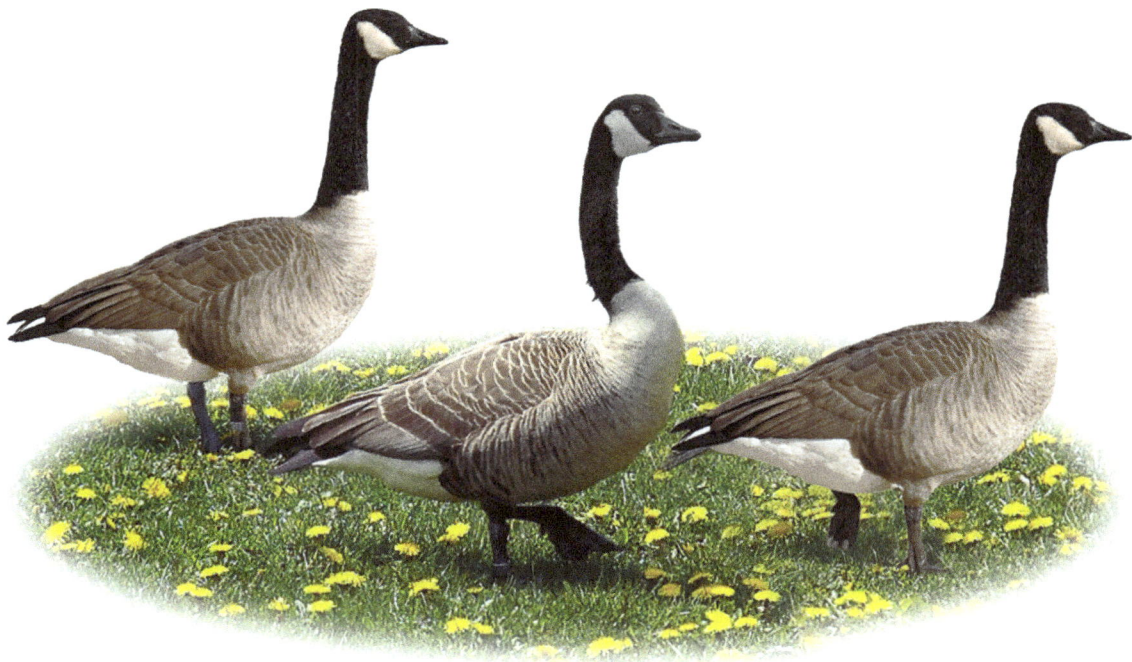

G – Initial Position

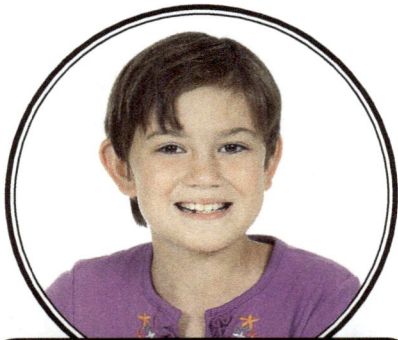

This is Gertrude. She gets all the things on this page.

1. Practice your sound by saying the words on this page. (Ex. geese, gears, etc.). Say the last word twice.

2. Practice saying **Gertrude** with each of the words. (Ex. Gertrude geese, Gertrude gears, etc.). Say the last word pair twice.

3. Practice saying **gets** with these words. (Ex. Gertrude gets geese, etc.). Say one of the sentences twice.

4. Practice saying **guilty** with these words. (Gertrude gets guilty geese, etc.). Say one of the expanded sentences twice.

When you have finished this whole page you will have said your sound in 100 words! Good job!

geese	gears	guest
guard	guide	guess
guarantee	goalie	gecko

U.S.D.A. PRIME
Satisfaction Guaranteed

Name _____

Helper Signature _____

Speech - Language Pathologist _____

Date _____

#BKCD-273 • *Say & Do® Artic Reps* • ©2015 Super Duper® Publications • www.superduperinc.com

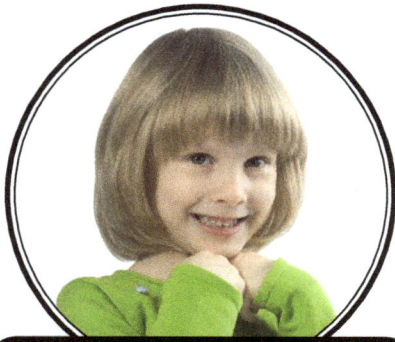

G – Initial Position

Gabby

This is Gabby. She gave all the things on this page.

1. Practice your sound by saying the words on this page. (Ex. gas, game, etc.). Say the last word twice.
2. Practice saying **Gabby** with each of the words. (Ex. Gabby gas, Gabby game, etc.). Say the last word pair twice.
3. Practice saying **gave** with these words. (Ex. Gabby gave gas etc.). Say one of the sentences twice.
4. Practice saying **gaudy** with these words. (Gabby gave gaudy gas, etc.). Say one of the expanded sentences twice.

When you have finished this whole page you will have said your sound in 100 words! Good job!

gas	game	garlic
gate	gadget	gallery
gallon	garage	garbage

Name _____

Speech - Language Pathologist _____

Helper Signature _____

Date _____

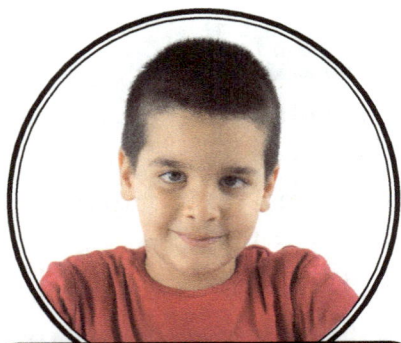

Gilbert

This is Gilbert. He gives all the things on this page.

G – Initial Position

1. Practice your sound by saying the words on this page. (Ex. gift, girl, etc.). Say the last word twice.

2. Practice saying **Gilbert** with each of the words. (Ex. Gilbert gift, Gilbert girl, etc.). Say the last word pair twice.

3. Practice saying **gives** with these words. (Ex. Gilbert gives a gift, etc.). Say one of the sentences twice.

4. Practice saying **gilded** with these words. (Gilbert gives a gilded gift, etc.). Say one of the expanded sentences twice.

When you have finished this whole page you will have said your sound in 100 words! Good job!

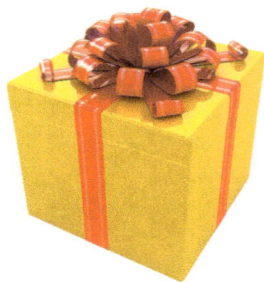 gift	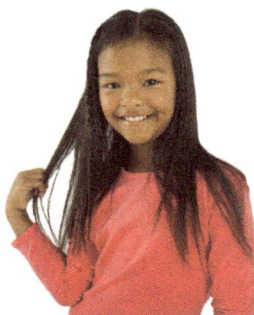 girl	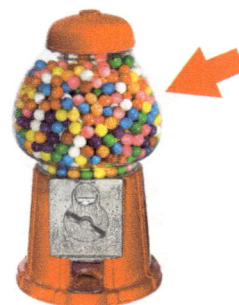 gumballs
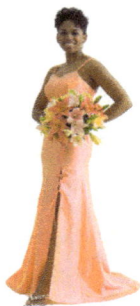 gown	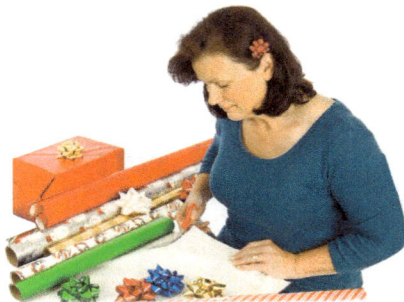 gift wrap	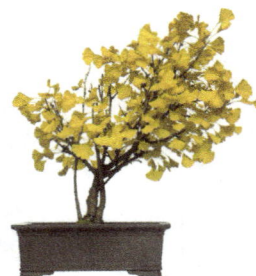 gingko
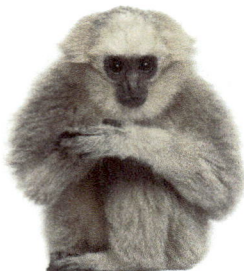 gibbon	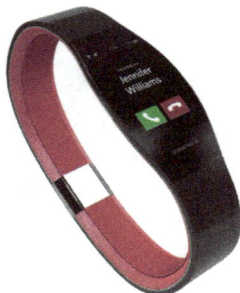 gizmo	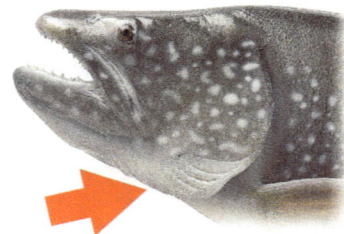 gill

Name

Speech - Language Pathologist

Helper Signature

Date

#BKCD-273 • *Say & Do® Artic Reps* • ©2015 Super Duper® Publications • www.superduperinc.com

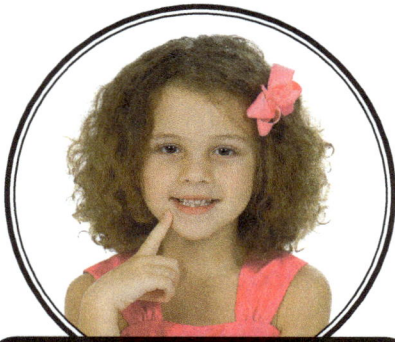

Goldie

This is Goldie. She goes to all the things on this page.

1. Practice your sound by saying the words on this page. (Ex. goal, gorilla, etc.). Say the last word twice.

2. Practice saying **Goldie** with each of the words. (Ex. Goldie goal, Goldie gorilla, etc.). Say the last word pair twice.

3. Practice saying **goes to** with these words. (Ex. Goldie goes to the goal, etc.). Say one of the sentences twice.

4. Practice saying **gooey** with these words. (Goldie goes to the gooey goal, etc.). Say one of the expanded sentences twice.

When you have finished this whole page you will have said your sound in 100 words! Good job!

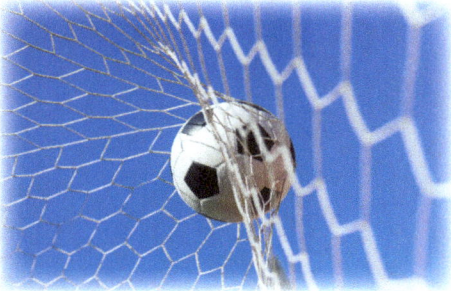 goal	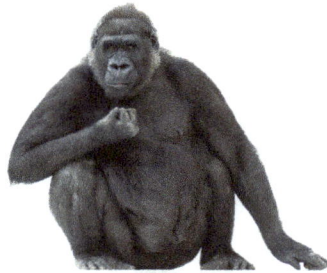 gorilla	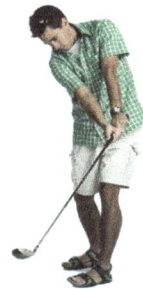 golf
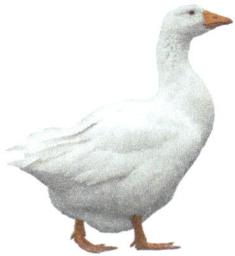 goose	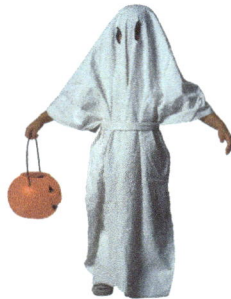 ghost	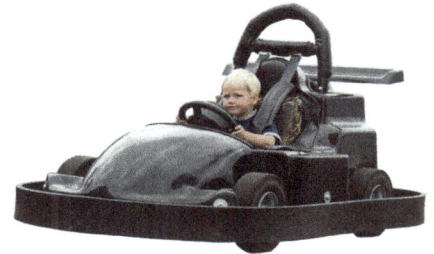 go-cart
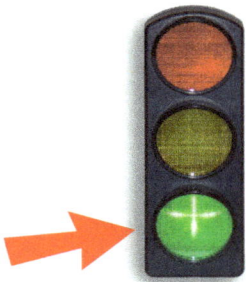 go	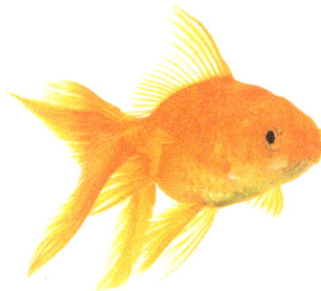 goldfish	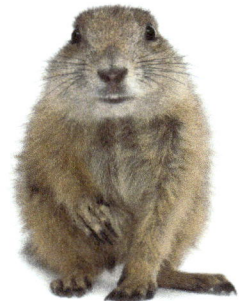 gopher

Name _____

Helper Signature _____

Speech - Language Pathologist _____

Date _____

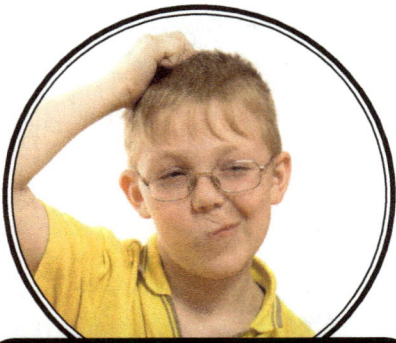

Gus

This is Gus. He guessed all the things on this page.

G – Initial Position

1. Practice your sound by saying the words on this page. (Ex. guppy, gumdrop, etc.). Say the last word twice.

2. Practice saying **Gus** with each of the words. (Ex. Gus guppy, Gus gumdrop, etc.). Say the last word pair twice.

3. Practice saying **guessed** with these words. (Ex. Gus guessed a guppy, etc.). Say one of the sentences twice.

4. Practice saying **gullible** with these words. (Gus guessed a gullible guppy, etc.). Say one of the expanded sentences twice.

When you have finished this whole page you will have said your sound in 100 words! Good job!

guppy	gumdrop	guitar
gull	gum	guy
gulf	gumbo	gully

Name

Speech - Language Pathologist

Helper Signature

Date

#BKCD-273 • *Say & Do® Artic Reps* • ©2015 Super Duper® Publications • www.superduperinc.com

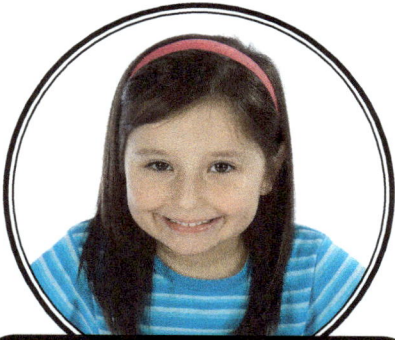

Maggie

This is Maggie. She was dragging all the things on this page.

G – Medial Position

1. Practice your sound by saying the words on this page. (Ex. dragon, alligator, etc.). Say the last word twice.
2. Practice saying **Maggie** with each of the words. (Ex. Maggie dragon, Maggie alligator, etc.). Say the last word pair twice.
3. Practice saying **was dragging** with these words. (Ex. Maggie was dragging a dragon, etc.). Say one of the sentences twice.
4. Practice saying **biggest** with these words. (Maggie was dragging the biggest dragon, etc.). Say one of the expanded sentences twice.

When you have finished this whole page you will have said your sound in 100 words! Good job!

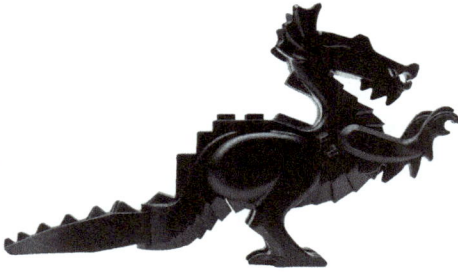

dragon

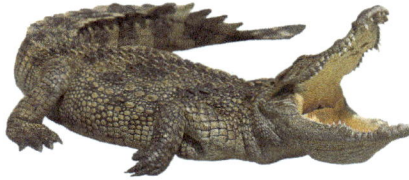

alligator

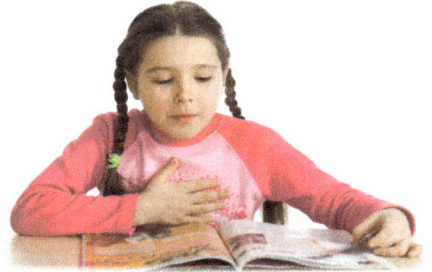

magazine

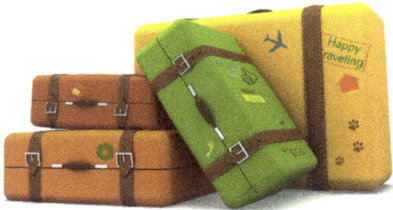

baggage

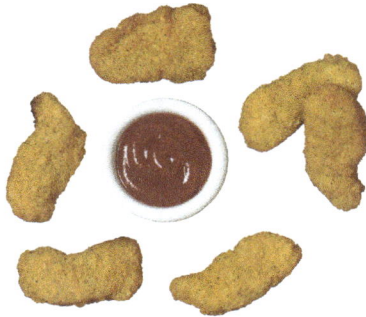

nuggets

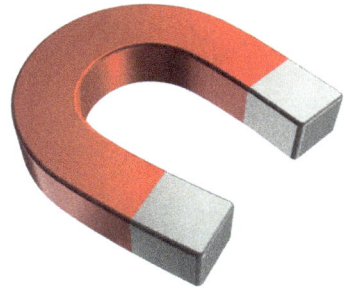

magnet

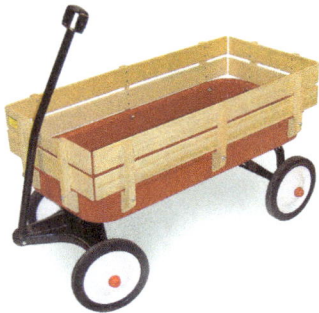

wagon

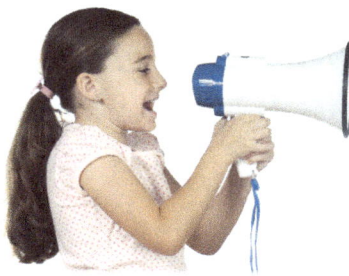

megaphone

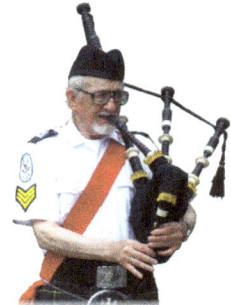

bagpipe

Name _____

Helper Signature _____

Speech - Language Pathologist _____

Date _____

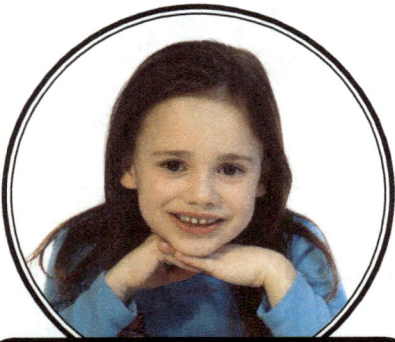

Peggy

This is Peggy. She was begging for things on this page.

1. Practice your sound by saying the words on this page. (Ex. buggy, dragonfly, etc.). Say the last word twice.

2. Practice saying **Peggy** with each of the words. (Ex. Peggy buggy, Peggy dragonfly, etc.). Say the last word pair twice.

3. Practice saying **was begging for** with these words. (Ex. Peggy was begging for a buggy, etc.). Say one of the sentences twice.

4. Practice saying **regular** with these words. (Peggy was begging for a regular buggy, etc.). Say one of the expanded sentences twice.

When you have finished this whole page you will have said your sound in 100 words! Good job!

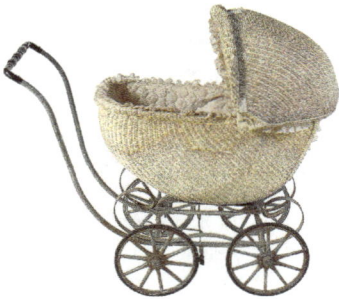 buggy	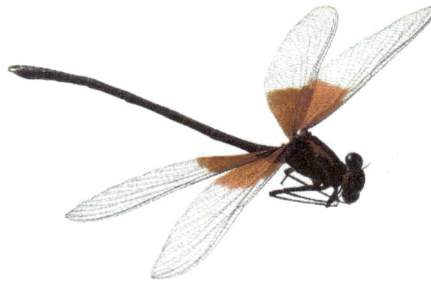 dragonfly	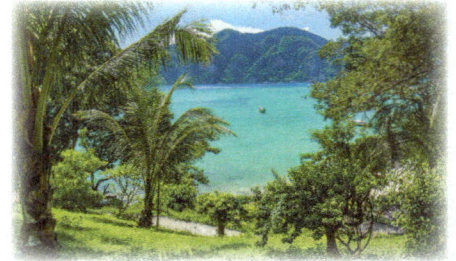 lagoon
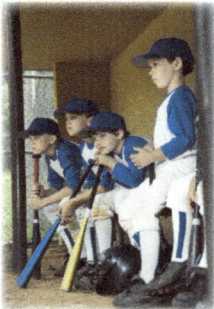 dugout	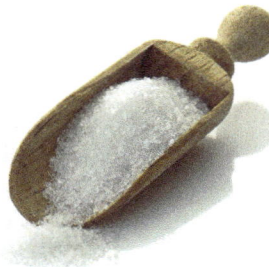 sugar	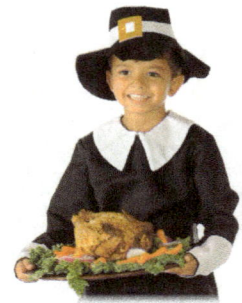 Thanksgiving
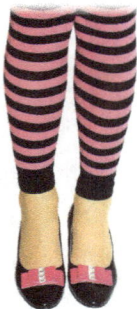 leggings	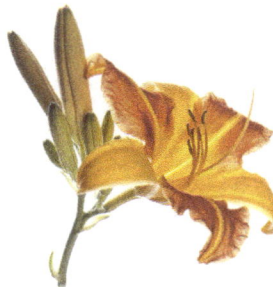 tiger lily	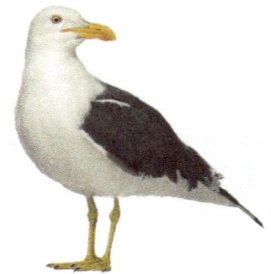 seagull

Name

Speech - Language Pathologist

Helper Signature

Date

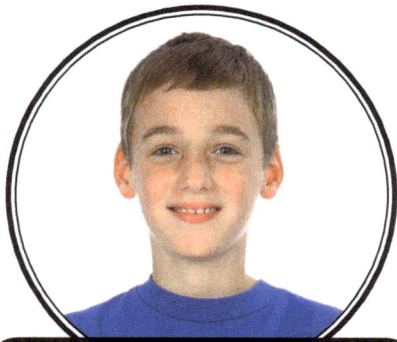

Iggy

This is Iggy. He was tagging all the things on this page.

G – Medial Position

1. Practice your sound by saying the words on this page. (Ex. tiger, cougar, etc.). Say the last word twice.

2. Practice saying **Iggy** with each of the words. (Ex. Iggy tiger, Iggy cougar, etc.). Say the last word pair twice.

3. Practice saying **was tagging** with these words. (Ex. Iggy was tagging the tiger etc.). Say one of the sentences twice.

4. Practice saying **disgusting** with these words. (Iggy was tagging the disgusting tiger, etc.). Say one of the expanded sentences twice.

When you have finished this whole page you will have said your sound in 100 words! Good job!

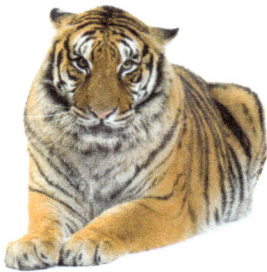 tiger	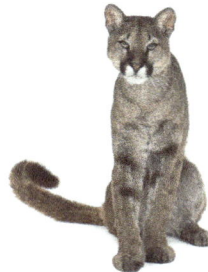 cougar	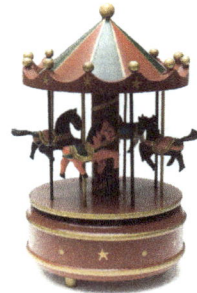 merry-go-round
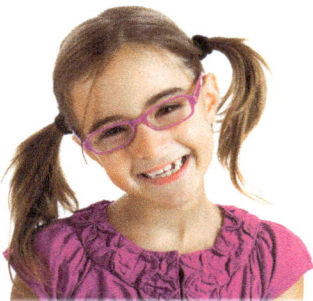 pigtail	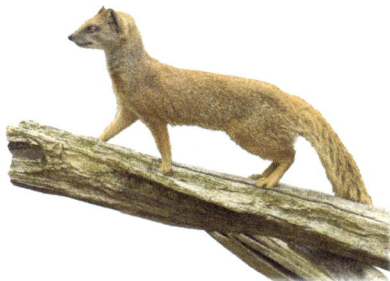 mongoose	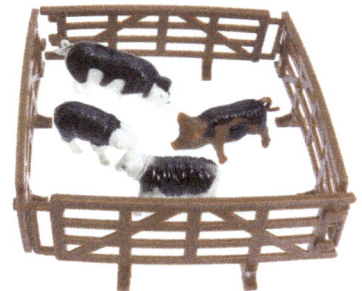 pigpen
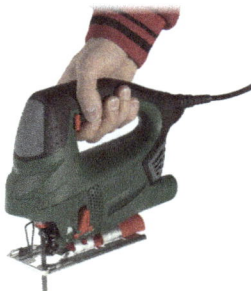 jigsaw	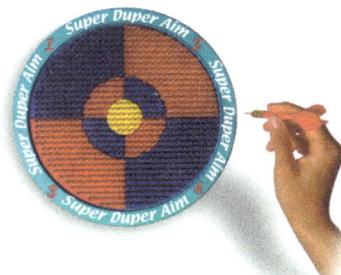 target	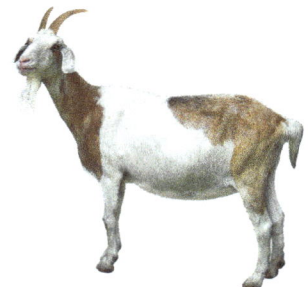 billy goat

Name _____

Helper Signature _____

Speech - Language Pathologist

Date

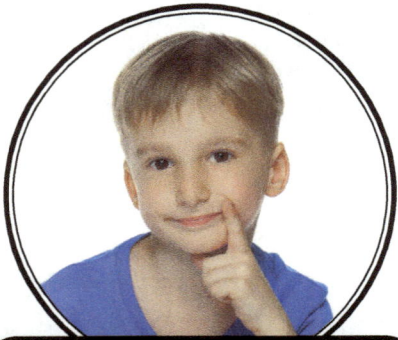

Logan

This is Logan. He is bagging all the things on this page.

G – Medial Position

1. Practice your sound by saying the words on this page. (Ex. luggage, hamburger, etc.). Say the last word twice.

2. Practice saying **Logan** with each of the words. (Ex. Logan luggage, Logan hamburger, etc.). Say the last word pair twice.

3. Practice saying **is bagging** with these words. (Ex. Logan is bagging luggage, etc.). Say one of the sentences twice.

4. Practice saying **elegant** with these words. (Logan is bagging elegant luggage, etc.). Say one of the expanded sentences twice.

When you have finished this whole page you will have said your sound in 100 words! Good job!

luggage	hamburger	tugboat
eggplant	doghouse	spaghetti
hot dogs	marigolds	pogo stick

Name _____

Helper Signature _____

Speech - Language Pathologist _____

Date _____

#BKCD-273 • *Say & Do*® Artic Reps • ©2015 Super Duper® Publications • www.superduperinc.com

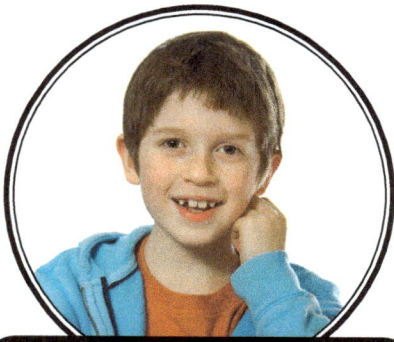

Doug

This is Doug. He will drag all the things on this page.

1. Practice your sound by saying the words on this page. (Ex. bag, flag, etc.). Say the last word twice.

2. Practice saying **Doug** with each of the words. (Ex. Doug bag, Doug flag, etc.). Say the last word pair twice.

3. Practice saying **will drag** with these words. (Ex. Doug will drag a bag, etc.). Say one of the sentences twice.

4. Practice saying **big** with these words. (Doug will drag a big bag, etc.). Say one of the expanded sentences twice.

When you have finished this whole page you will have said your sound in 100 words! Good job!

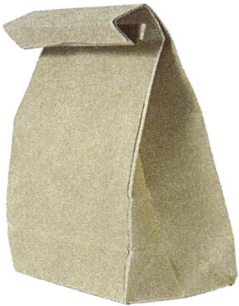 bag	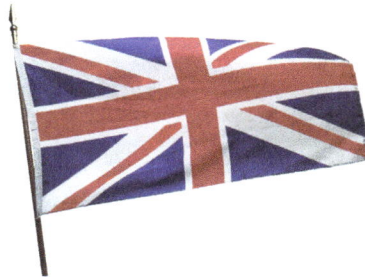 flag	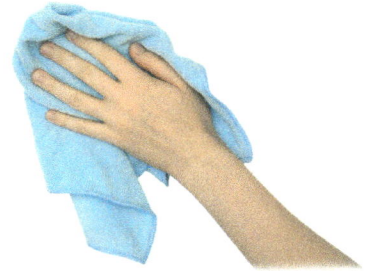 rag
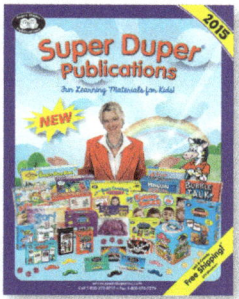 catalog	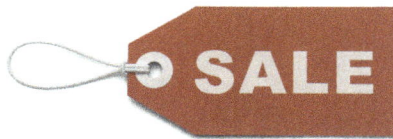 tag	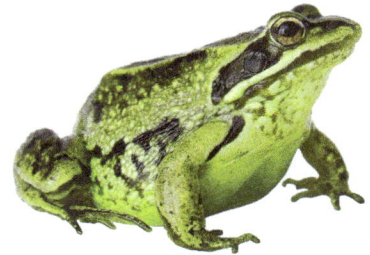 frog
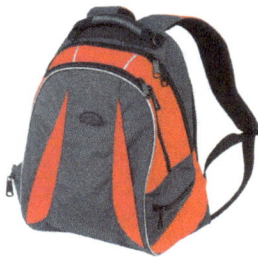 bookbag	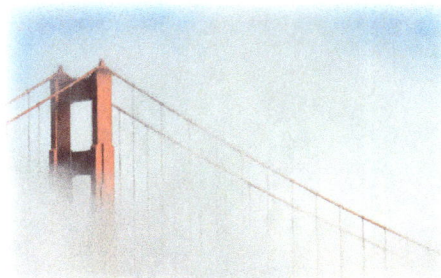 fog	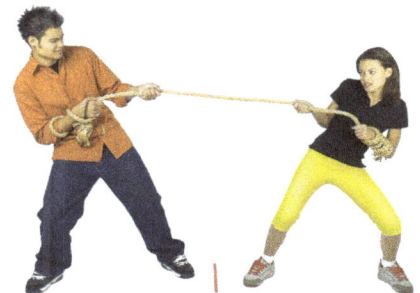 tug

Name _____

Helper Signature _____

Speech - Language Pathologist _____

Date _____

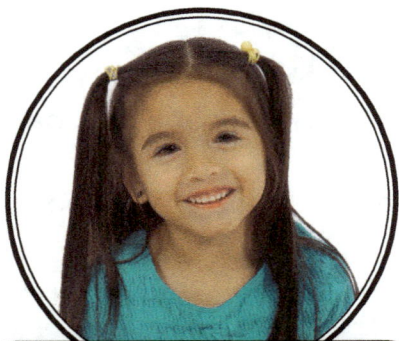

Meg

This is Meg. She will beg for all the things on this page.

G – Final Position

1. Practice your sound by saying the words on this page. (Ex. dog, groundhog, etc.). Say the last word twice.

2. Practice saying **Meg** with each of the words. (Ex. Meg dog, Meg groundhog, etc.). Say the last word pair twice.

3. Practice saying **will beg for** with these words. (Ex. Meg will beg for a dog, etc.). Say one of the sentences twice.

4. Practice saying **snug** with these words. (Meg will beg for a snug dog, etc.). Say one of the expanded sentences twice.

When you have finished this whole page you will have said your sound in 100 words! Good job!

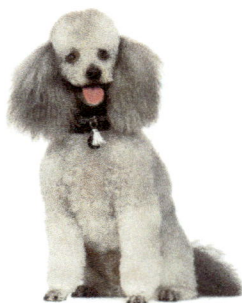 dog	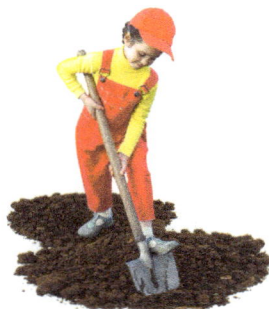 dig	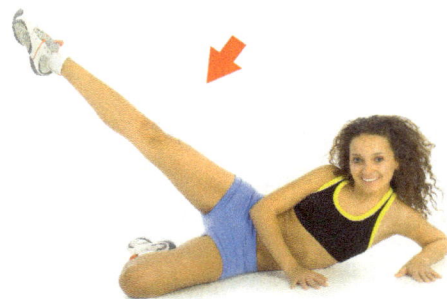 leg
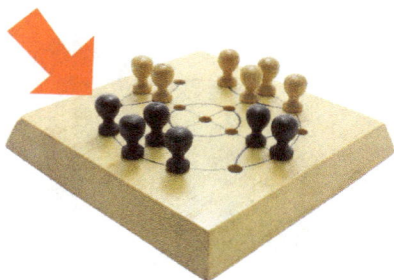 peg	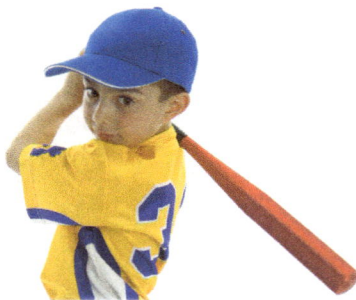 little league	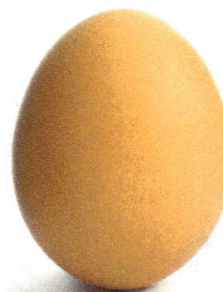 egg
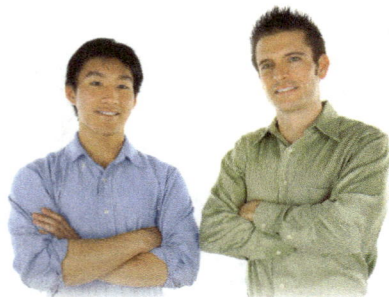 colleague	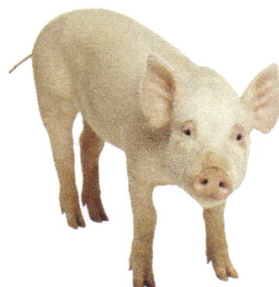 hog	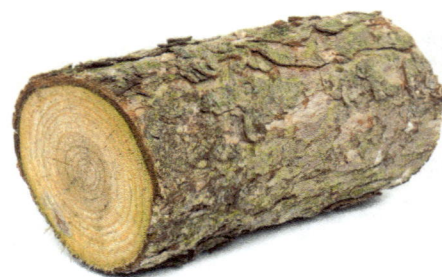 log

Name _____

Helper Signature _____

Speech - Language Pathologist _____

Date _____

#BKCD-273 • *Say & Do® Artic Reps* • ©2015 Super Duper® Publications • www.superduperinc.com

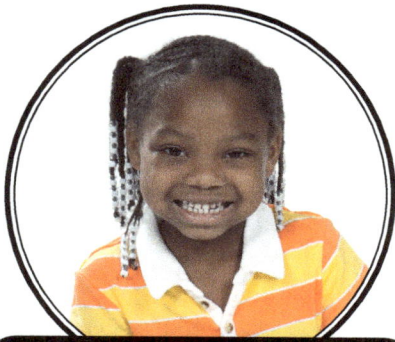

Peg

This is Peg. She will hug all the things on this page.

G – Final Position

1. Practice your sound by saying the words on this page. (Ex. stag, fig, etc.). Say the last word twice.

2. Practice saying **Peg** with each of the words. (Ex. Peg stag, Peg fig etc.). Say the last word pair twice.

3. Practice saying **will hug** with these words. (Ex. Peg will hug a stag, etc.). Say one of the sentences twice.

4. Practice saying **big** with these words. (Peg will hug a big stag, etc.). Say one of the expanded sentences twice.

   When you have finished this whole page you will have said your sound in 100 words! Good job!

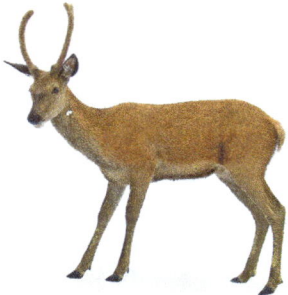 stag	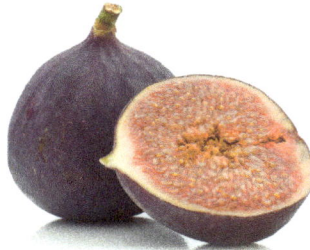 fig	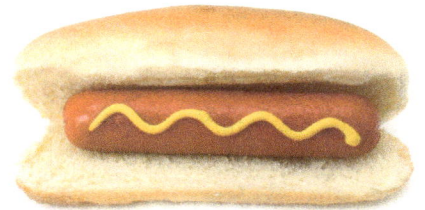 hot dog
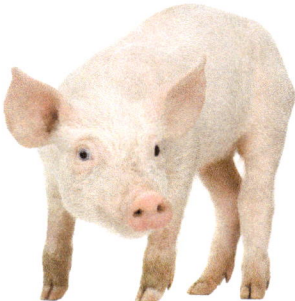 pig	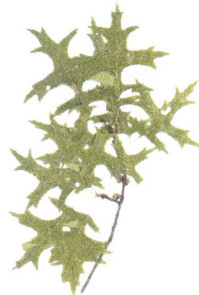 twig	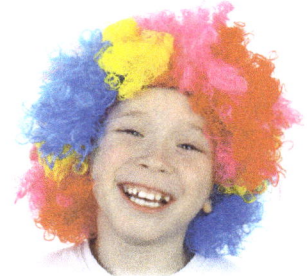 wig
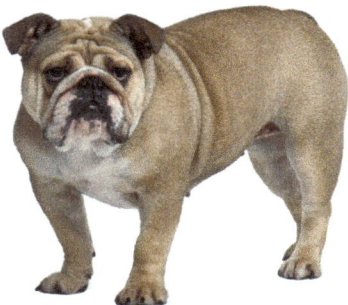 bulldog	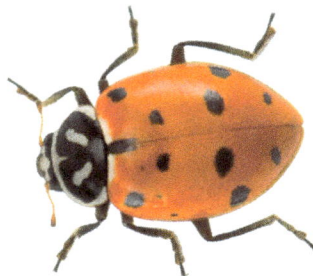 ladybug	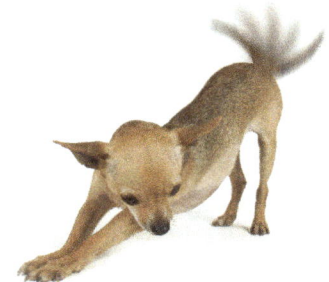 wag

Name _____

Helper Signature _____

Speech - Language Pathologist _____

Date _____

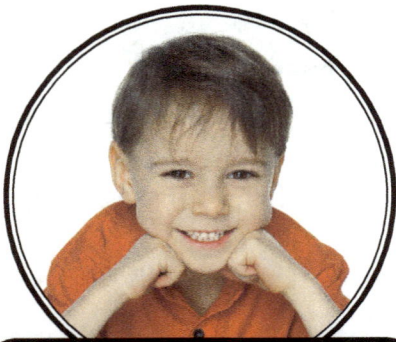

Craig

This is Craig. He dug for all the things on this page.

G – Final Position

1. Practice your sound by saying the words on this page. (Ex. bug, jug, etc.). Say the last word twice.

2. Practice saying **Craig** with each of the words. (Ex. Craig bug, Craig jug etc.). Say the last word pair twice.

3. Practice saying **dug for** with these words. (Ex. Craig dug for a bug, etc.). Say one of the sentences twice.

4. Practice saying **smug** with these words. (Craig dug for a smug bug, etc.). Say one of the expanded sentences twice.

When you have finished this whole page you will have said your sound in 100 words! Good job!

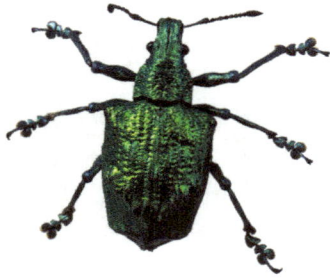	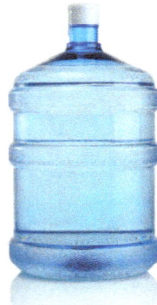	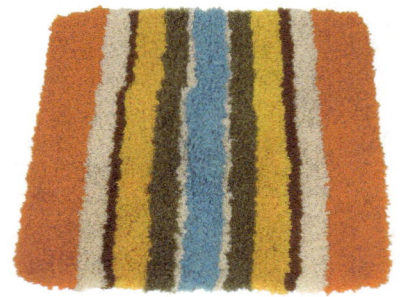
bug	jug	rug
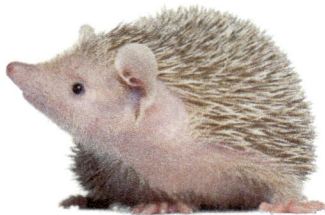	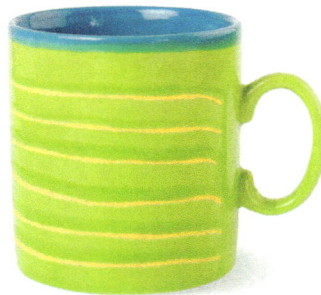	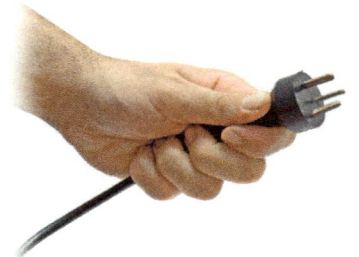
hedgehog	mug	plug
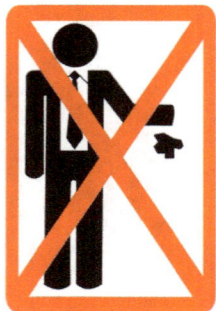	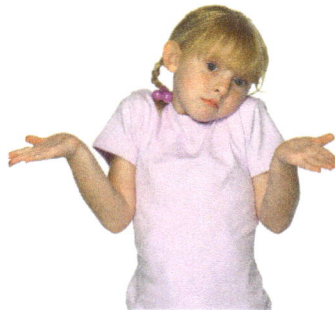	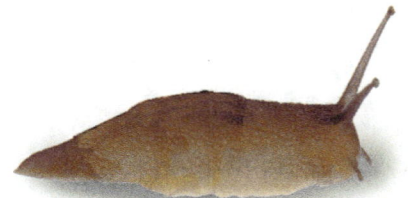
litterbug	shrug	slug

Name _____

Helper Signature _____

Speech - Language Pathologist _____

Date _____

#BKCD-273 • *Say & Do® Artic Reps* • ©2015 Super Duper® Publications • www.superduperinc.com

K

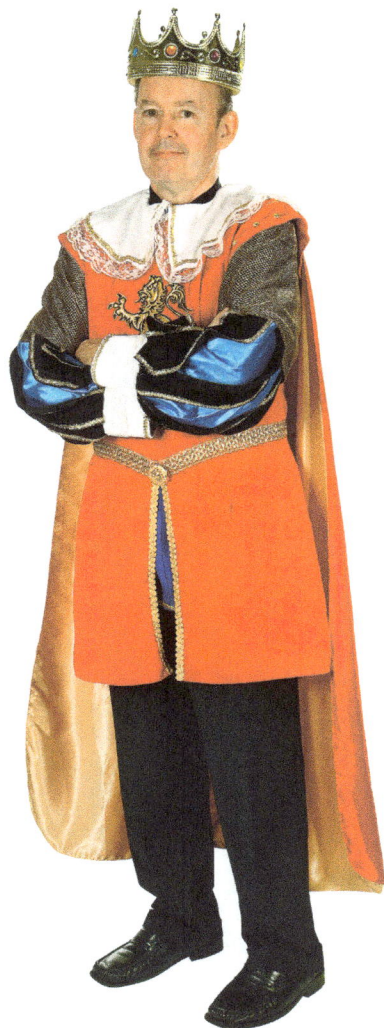

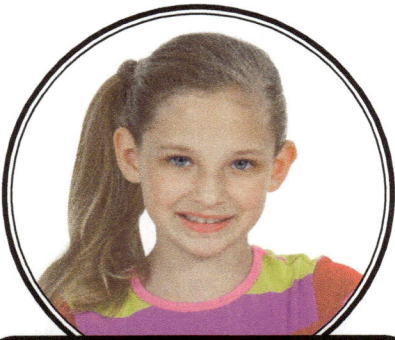

Kay

This is Kay. She carried all the things on this page.

1. Practice your sound by saying the words on this page. (Ex. candle, caramels, etc.). Say the last word twice.

2. Practice saying **Kay** with each of the words. (Ex. Kay candle, Kay caramels, etc.). Say the last word pair twice.

3. Practice saying **carried** with these words. (Ex. Kay carried a candle, etc.). Say one of the sentences twice.

4. Practice saying **canvas** with these words. (Kay carried a canvas candle, etc.). Say one of the expanded sentences twice.

When you have finished this whole page you will have said your sound in 100 words! Good job!

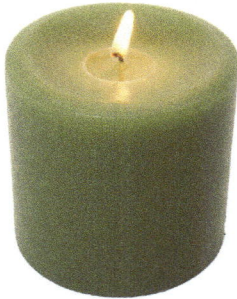 candle	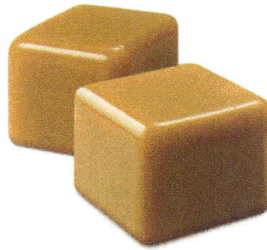 caramels	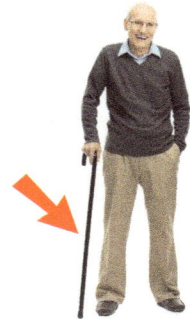 cane
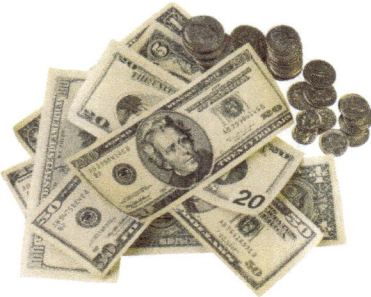 cash	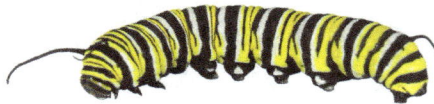 caterpillar	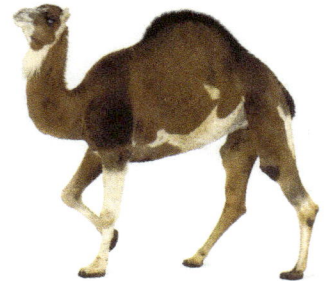 camel
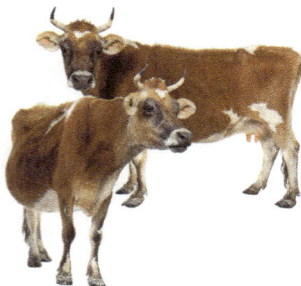 cattle	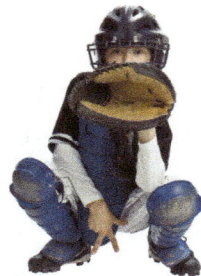 catcher	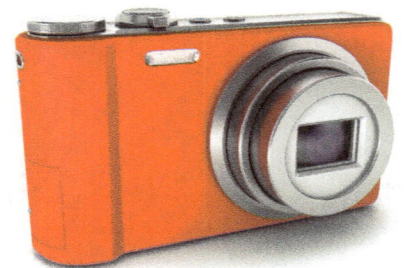 camera

Name _____

Helper Signature _____

Speech - Language Pathologist _____

Date _____

#BKCD-273 • *Say & Do® Artic Reps* • ©2015 Super Duper® Publications • www.superduperinc.com

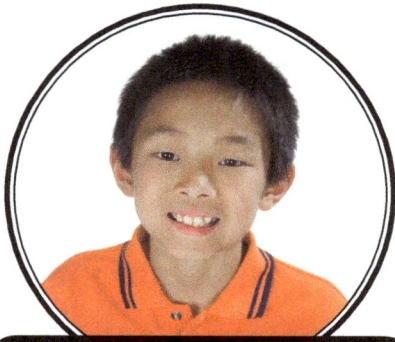

Kevin

This is Kevin. He keeps all the things on this page.

K – Initial Position

1. Practice your sound by saying the words on this page. (Ex. key, kettle, etc.). Say the last word twice.

2. Practice saying **Kevin** with each of the words. (Ex. Kevin key, Kevin kettle, etc.). Say the last word pair twice.

3. Practice saying **keeps** with these words. (Ex. Kevin keeps the key, etc.). Say one of the sentences twice.

4. Practice saying **keen** with these words. (Kevin keeps a keen key, etc.). Say one of the expanded sentences twice.

When you have finished this whole page you will have said your sound in 100 words! Good job!

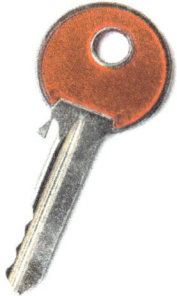 key	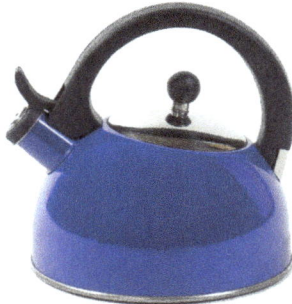 kettle	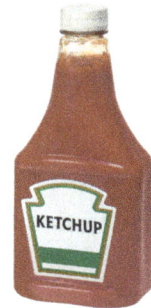 ketchup
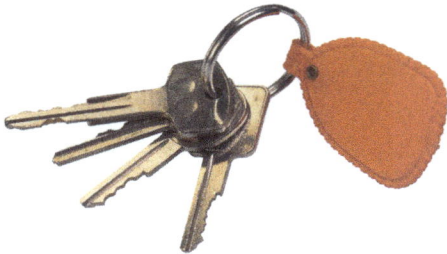 key chain	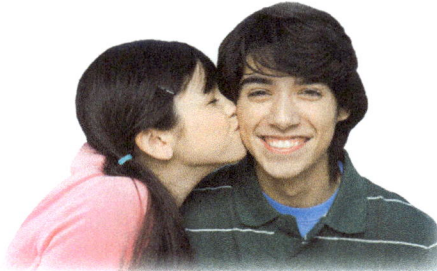 kiss	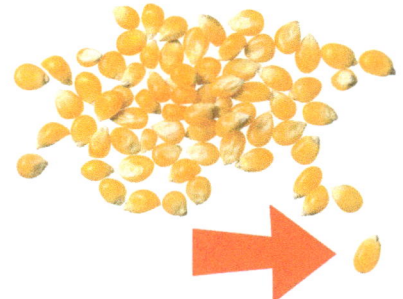 kernel
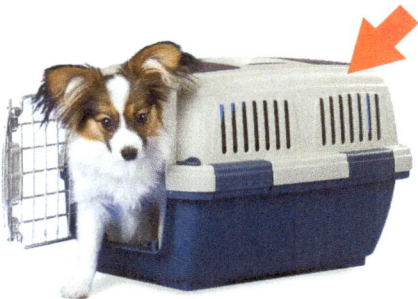 kennel	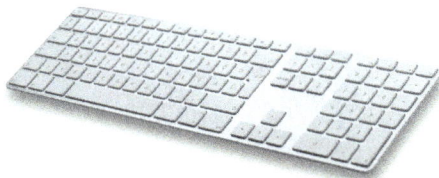 keyboard	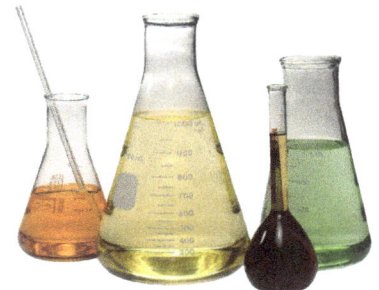 chemistry

Name _____

Helper Signature _____

Speech - Language Pathologist

Date

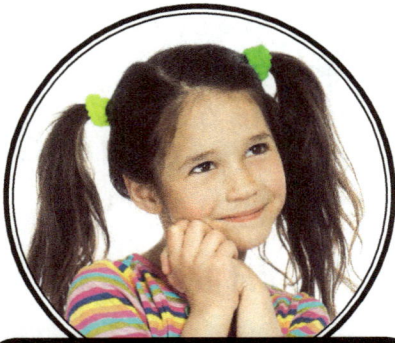

Kim

This is Kim. She kissed all the things on this page.

K – Initial Position

1. Practice your sound by saying the words on this page. (Ex. kids, king, etc.). Say the last word twice.

2. Practice saying **Kim** with each of the words. (Ex. Kim kids, Kim king, etc.). Say the last word pair twice.

3. Practice saying **kissed** with these words. (Ex. Kim kissed the kids, etc.). Say one of the sentences twice.

4. Practice saying **kind** with these words. (Kim kissed the kind kids, etc.). Say one of the expanded sentences twice.

When you have finished this whole page you will have said your sound in 100 words! Good job!

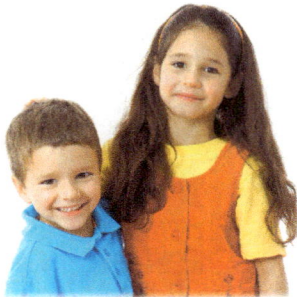 kids	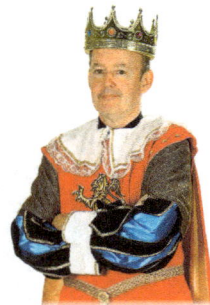 king	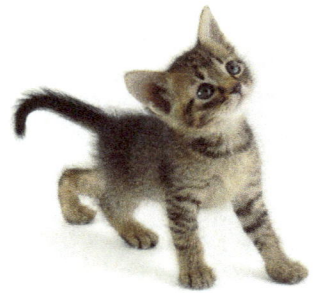 kitten
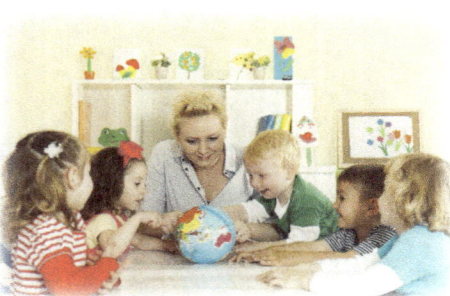 kindergarten	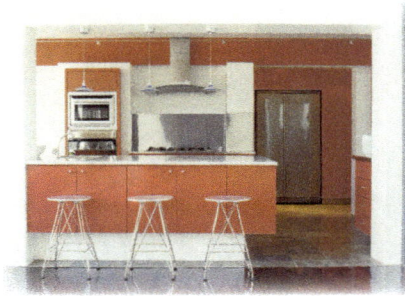 kitchen	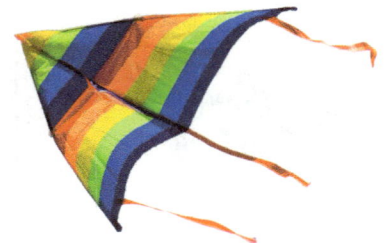 kite
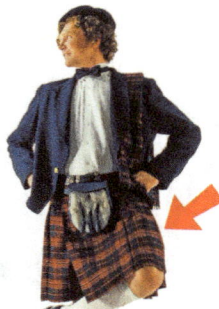 kilt	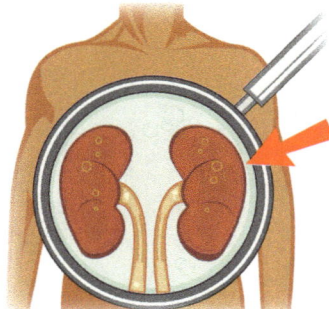 kidney	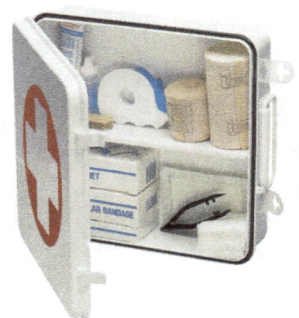 kit

Name _____

Helper Signature _____

Speech - Language Pathologist _____

Date _____

#BKCD-273 • *Say & Do® Artic Reps* • ©2015 Super Duper® Publications • www.superduperinc.com

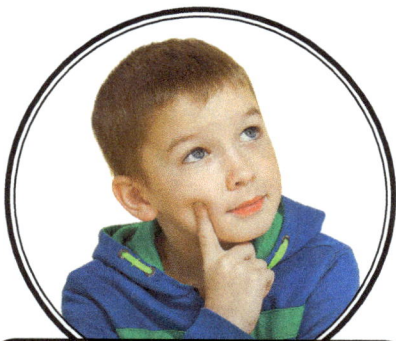

Cody

This is Cody. He counts all the things on this page.

1. Practice your sound by saying the words on this page. (Ex. combs, coats, etc.). Say the last word twice.

2. Practice saying **Cody** with each of the words. (Ex. Cody combs, Cody coats, etc.). Say the last word pair twice.

3. Practice saying **counts** with these words. (Ex. Cody counts combs, etc.). Say one of the sentences twice.

4. Practice saying **cool** with these words. (Cody counts cool combs, etc.). Say one of the expanded sentences twice.

When you have finished this whole page you will have said your sound in 100 words! Good job!

combs	coats	coins
candy	couches	cowboys
cobras	corn	cones

Name _____

Speech - Language Pathologist _____

Helper Signature _____

Date _____

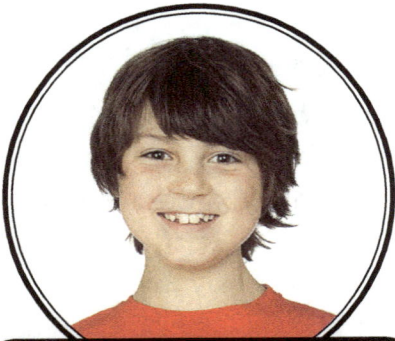

Curt

This is Curt. He cuts all the things on this page.

K – Initial Position

1. Practice your sound by saying the words on this page. (Ex. cushion, canoes, etc.). Say the last word twice.

2. Practice saying **Curt** with each of the words. (Ex. Curt cushion, Curt canoes, etc.). Say the last word pair twice.

3. Practice saying **cuts** with these words. (Ex. Curt cuts the cushion, etc.). Say one of the sentences twice.

4. Practice saying **cute** with these words. (Curt cuts a cute cushion, etc.). Say one of the expanded sentences twice.

When you have finished this whole page you will have said your sound in 100 words! Good job!

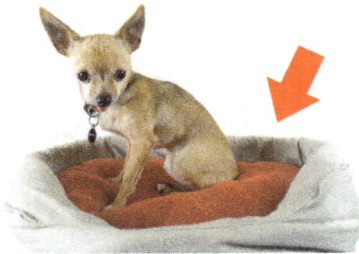 cushion	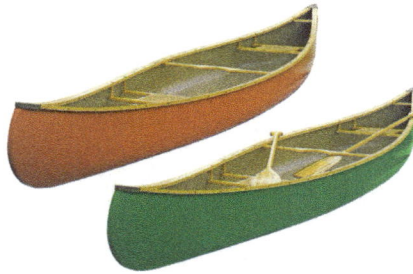 canoes	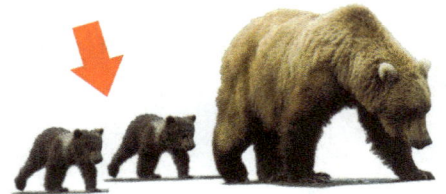 cubs
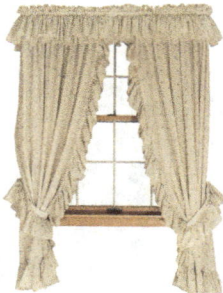 curtains	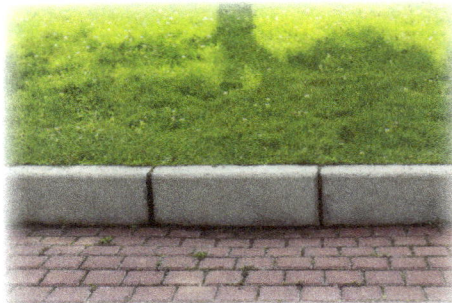 curb	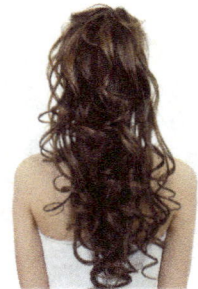 curl
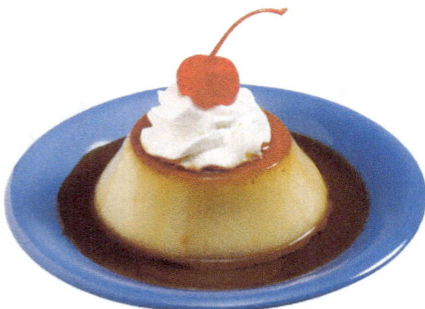 custard	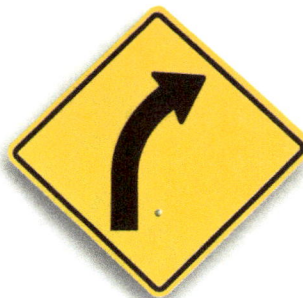 curve	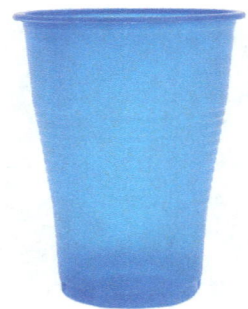 cup

Name _____

Helper Signature _____

Speech - Language Pathologist _____

Date _____

#BKCD-273 • *Say & Do® Artic Reps* • ©2015 Super Duper® Publications • www.superduperinc.com

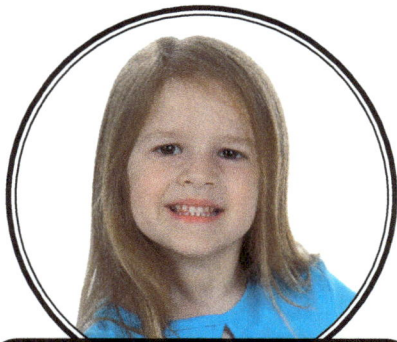

Jackie

This is Jackie. She was making all the things on this page.

K – Medial Position

1. Practice your sound by saying the words on this page. (Ex. bacon, jacket, etc.). Say the last word twice.

2. Practice saying **Jackie** with each of the words. (Ex. Jackie bacon, Jackie jacket, etc.). Say the last word pair twice.

3. Practice saying **was making** with these words. (Ex. Jackie was making bacon, etc.). Say one of the sentences twice.

4. Practice saying **delicate** with these words. (Jackie was making delicate bacon, etc.). Say one of the expanded sentences twice.

When you have finished this whole page you will have said your sound in 100 words! Good job!

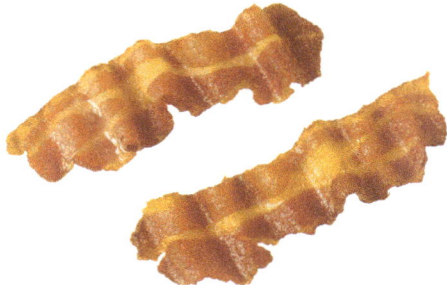 bacon	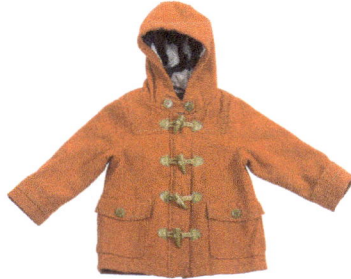 jacket	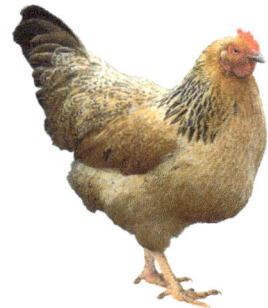 chicken
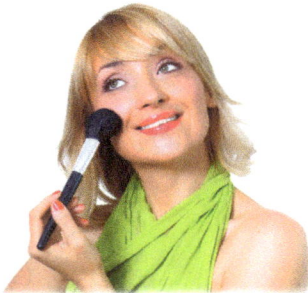 makeup	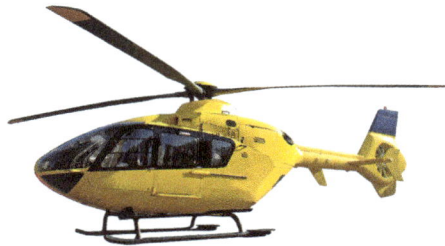 helicopter	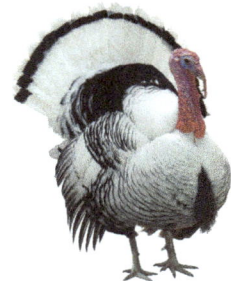 turkey
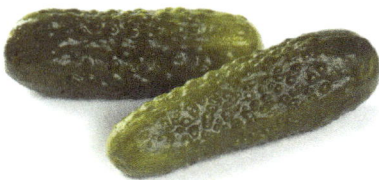 pickles	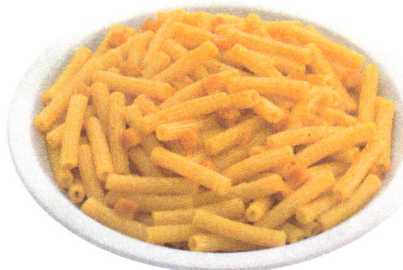 macaroni	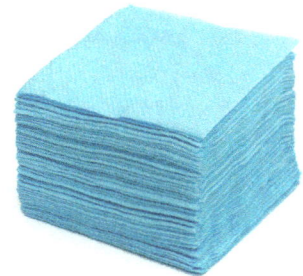 napkin

Name _____

Helper Signature _____

Speech - Language Pathologist _____

Date _____

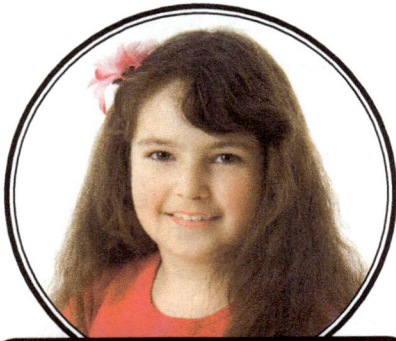

Becky

This is Becky. She was packing all the things on this page.

K – Medial Position

1. Practice your sound by saying the words on this page. (Ex. locket, mannequin, etc.). Say the last word twice.

2. Practice saying **Becky** with each of the words. (Ex. Becky locket, Becky mannequin, etc.). Say the last word pair twice.

3. Practice saying **was packing** with these words. (Ex. Becky was packing a locket, etc.). Say one of the sentences twice.

4. Practice saying **broken** with these words. (Becky was packing a broken locket, etc.). Say one of the expanded sentences twice.

When you have finished this whole page you will have said your sound in 100 words! Good job!

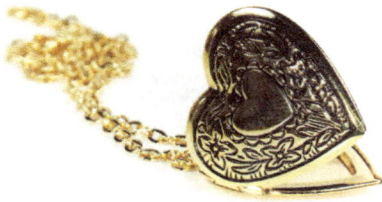

locket

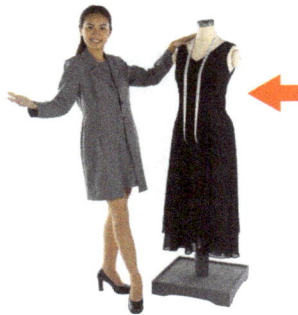

mannequin

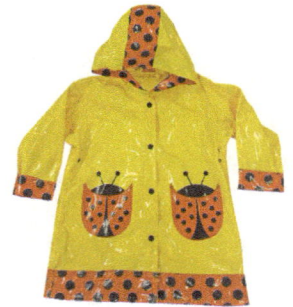

raincoat

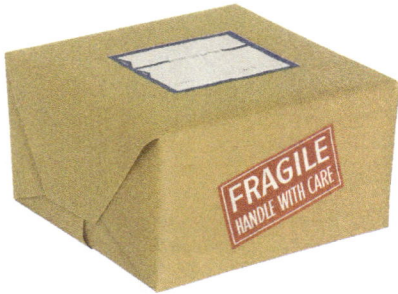

package

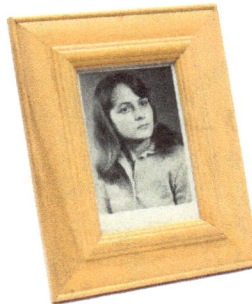

picture

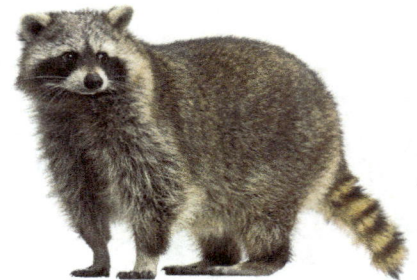

raccoon

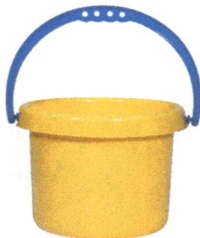

bucket

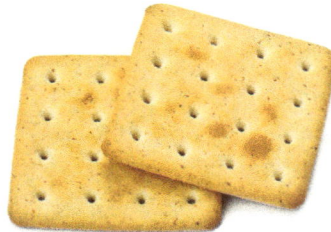

crackers

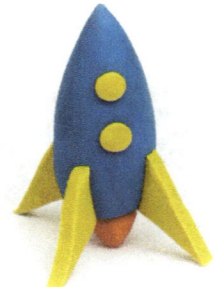

rocket

Name

Speech - Language Pathologist

Helper Signature

Date

#BKCD-273 • *Say & Do*® Artic Reps • ©2015 Super Duper® Publications • www.superduperinc.com

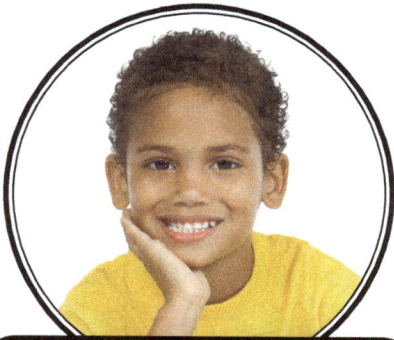

Mickey

This is Mickey. He was picking up things on this page.

K – Medial Position

1. Practice your sound by saying the words on this page. (Ex. monkey, bookcase, etc.). Say the last word twice.

2. Practice saying **Mickey** with each of the words. (Ex. Mickey monkey, Mickey bookcase, etc.). Say the last word pair twice.

3. Practice saying **was picking up** with these words. (Ex. Mickey was picking up the monkey, etc.). Say one of the sentences twice.

4. Practice saying **lucky** with these words. (Mickey was picking up a lucky monkey, etc.). Say one of the expanded sentences twice.

When you have finished this whole page you will have said your sound in 100 words! Good job!

monkey	bookcase	acorns
sneakers	checkers	coconut
America	side car	lockers

Name

Speech - Language Pathologist

Helper Signature

Date

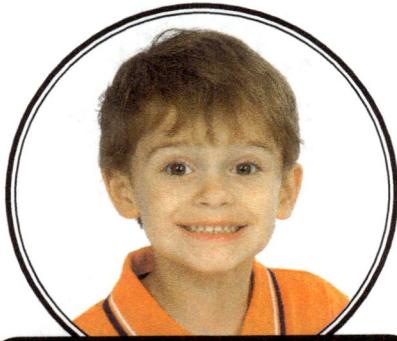

Chucky

This is Chucky. He was looking at at all the things on this page.

K – Medial Position

1. Practice your sound by saying the words on this page. (Ex. bobcat, donkey, etc.). Say the last word twice.
2. Practice saying **Chucky** with each of the words. (Ex. Chucky bobcat, Chucky donkey, etc.). Say the last word pair twice.
3. Practice saying **was looking at** with these words. (Ex. Chucky was looking at a bobcat, etc.). Say one of the sentences twice.
4. Practice saying **sticky** with these words. (Chucky was looking at a sticky bobcat, etc.). Say one of the expanded sentences twice.

When you have finished this whole page you will have said your sound in 100 words! Good job!

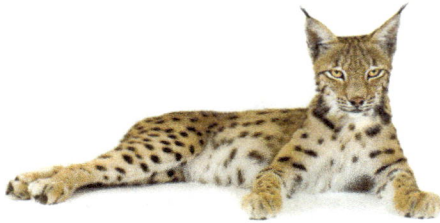 bobcat	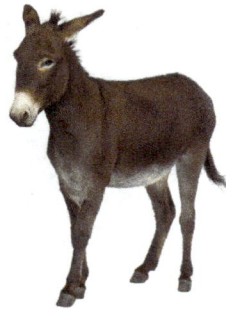 donkey	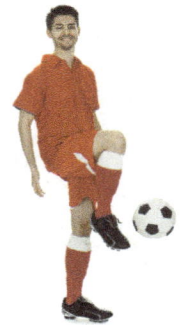 soccer
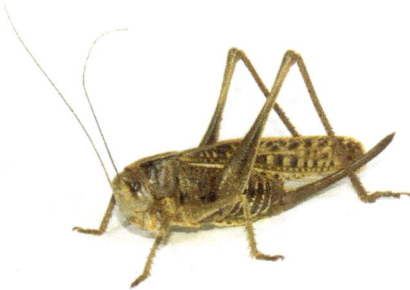 locust	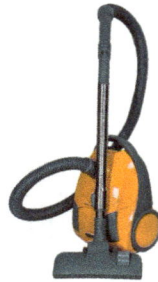 vacuum	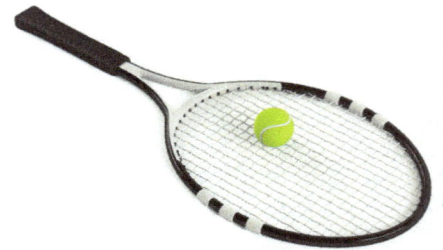 racket
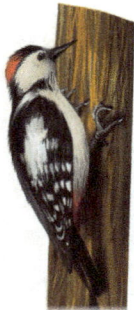 woodpecker	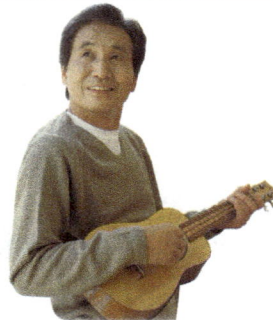 ukulele	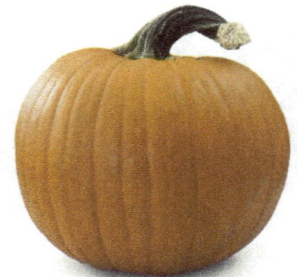 pumpkin

Name _____

Helper Signature _____

Speech - Language Pathologist _____

Date _____

#BKCD-273 • *Say & Do® Artic Reps* • ©2015 Super Duper® Publications • www.superduperinc.com

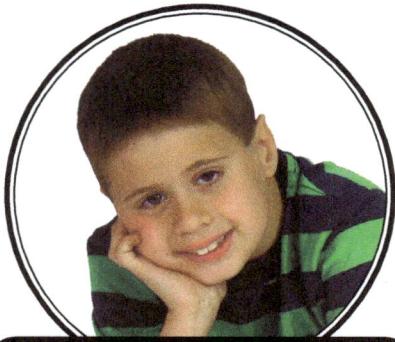

Jack

This is Jack. He took all the things on this page.

K – Final Position

1. Practice your sound by saying the words on this page. (Ex. snake, beak, etc.). Say the last word twice.

2. Practice saying **Jack** with each of the words. (Ex. Jack snake, Jack beak, etc.). Say the last word pair twice.

3. Practice saying **took** with these words. (Ex. Jack took a snake, etc.). Say one of the sentences twice.

4. Practice saying **black** with these words. (Jack took a black snake, etc.). Say one of the expanded sentences twice.

When you have finished this whole page you will have said your sound in 100 words! Good job!

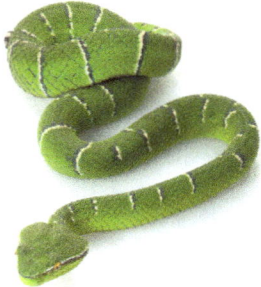 snake	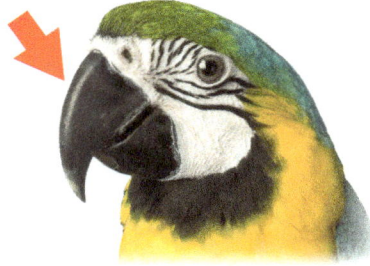 beak	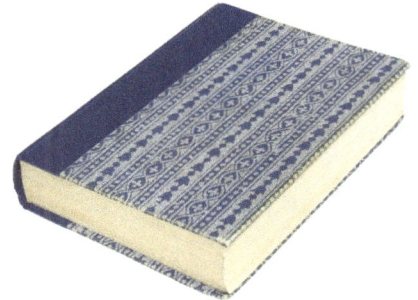 book
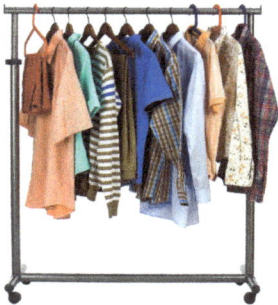 rack	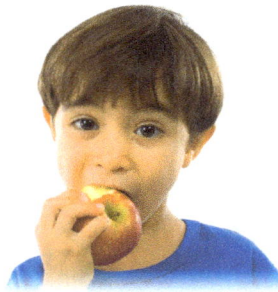 snack	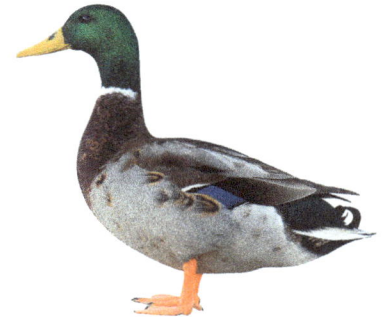 duck
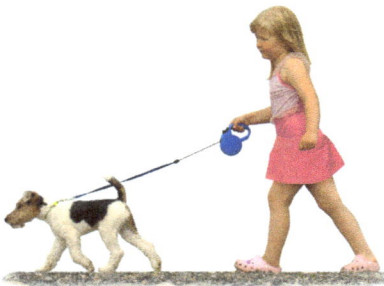 walk	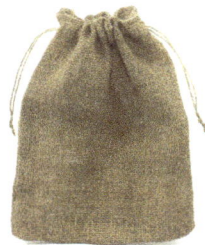 sack	 black

Name _____

Helper Signature _____

Speech - Language Pathologist _____

Date _____

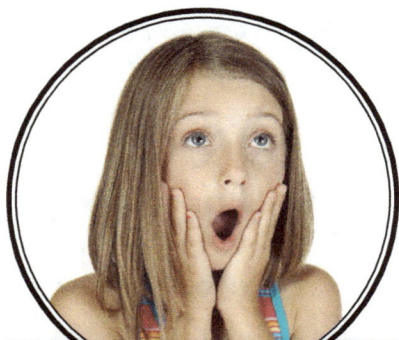

Brooke

This is Brooke. She shook all the things on this page.

1. Practice your sound by saying the words on this page. (Ex. sock, steak, etc.). Say the last word twice.

2. Practice saying **Brooke** with each of the words. (Ex. Brooke sock, Brooke steak, etc.). Say the last word pair twice.

3. Practice saying **shook** with these words. (Ex. Brooke shook a sock, etc.). Say one of the sentences twice.

4. Practice saying **meek** with these words. (Brooke shook a meek sock, etc.). Say one of the expanded sentences twice.

   When you have finished this whole page you will have said your sound in 100 words! Good job!

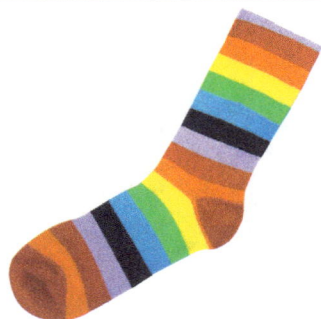

sock

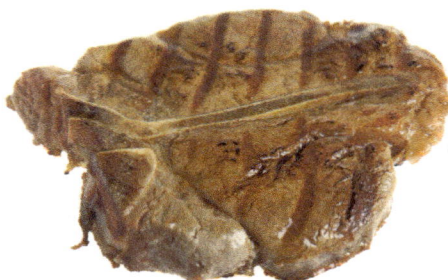

steak

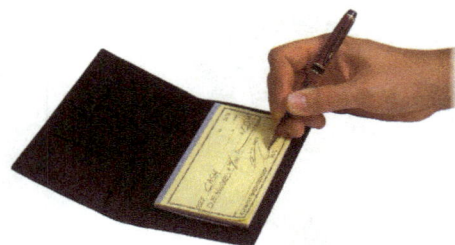

check

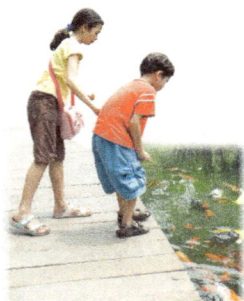

dock

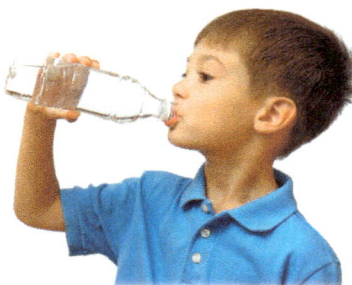

drink

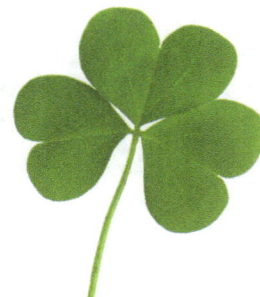

shamrock

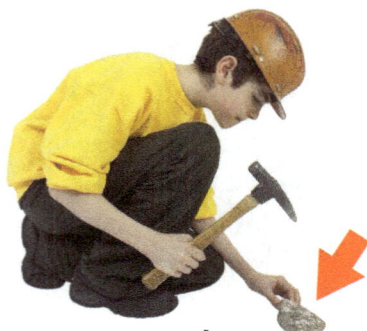

rock

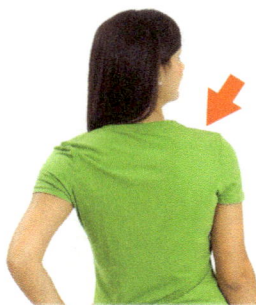

back

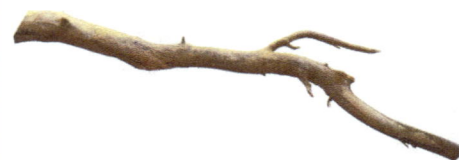

stick

Name

Helper Signature

Speech - Language Pathologist

Date

#BKCD-273 • Say & Do® Artic Reps • ©2015 Super Duper® Publications • www.superduperinc.com

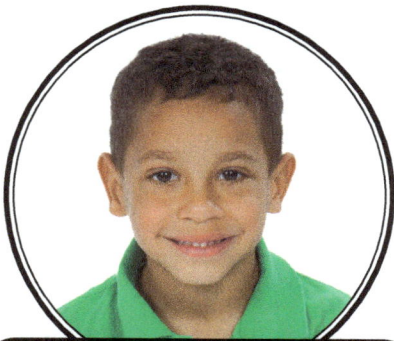

Mike

This is Mike. He broke all the things on this page.

K – Final Position

1. Practice your sound by saying the words on this page. (Ex. lock, chalk, etc.). Say the last word twice.

2. Practice saying **Mike** with each of the words. (Ex. Mike lock, Mike chalk, etc.). Say the last word pair twice.

3. Practice saying **broke** with these words. (Ex. Mike broke the lock, etc.). Say one of the sentences twice.

4. Practice saying **thick** with these words. (Mike broke a thick lock, etc.). Say one of the expanded sentences twice.

When you have finished this whole page you will have said your sound in 100 words! Good job!

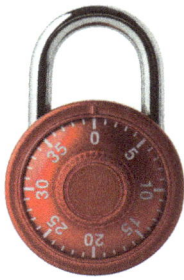 lock	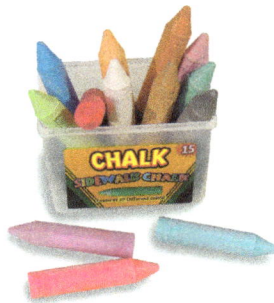 chalk	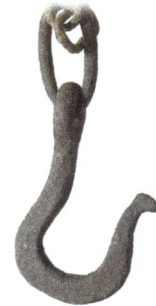 hook
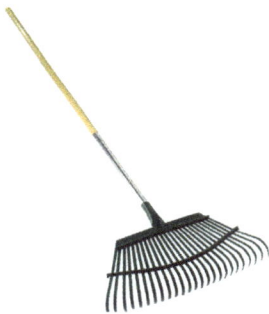 rake	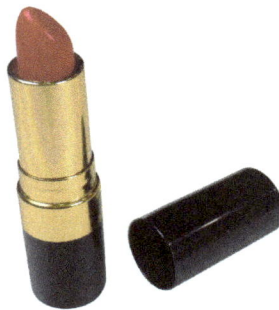 lipstick	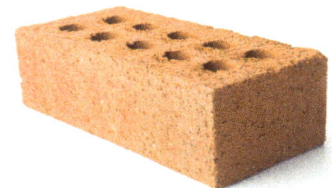 brick
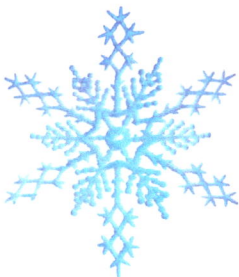 snowflake	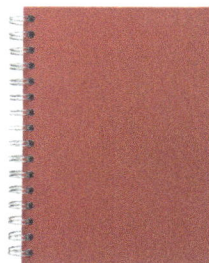 notebook	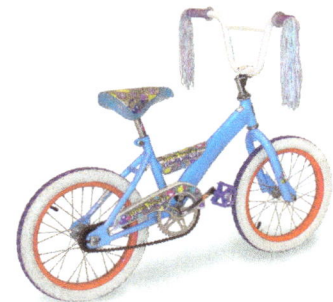 bike

Name _____

Helper Signature _____

Speech - Language Pathologist _____

Date _____

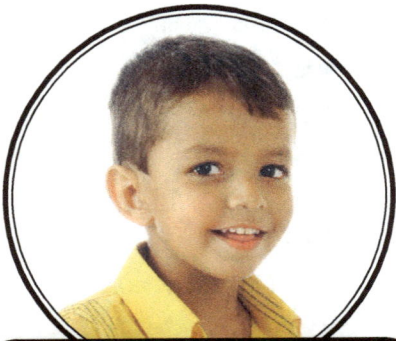

Duke

This is Duke. He will walk to all the things on this page.

K – Final Position

1. Practice your sound by saying the words on this page. (Ex. cook, phone book, etc.). Say the last word twice.

2. Practice saying **Duke** with each of the words. (Ex. Duke pack, Duke phone book, etc.). Say the last word pair twice.

3. Practice saying **will walk to** with these words. (Ex. Duke will walk to pack, etc.). Say one of the sentences twice.

4. Practice saying **plastic** with these words. (Duke will walk to a plastic pack, etc.). Say one of the expanded sentences twice.

When you have finished this whole page you will have said your sound in 100 words! Good job!

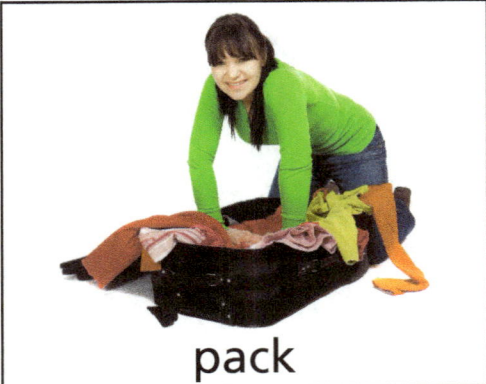 pack	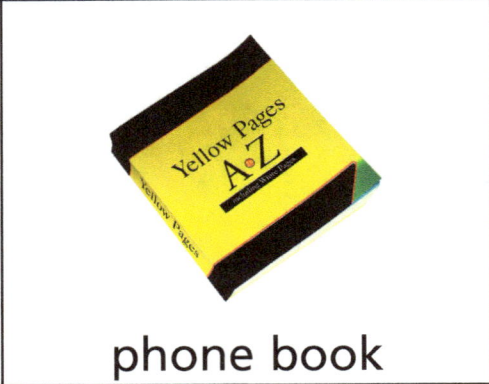 phone book	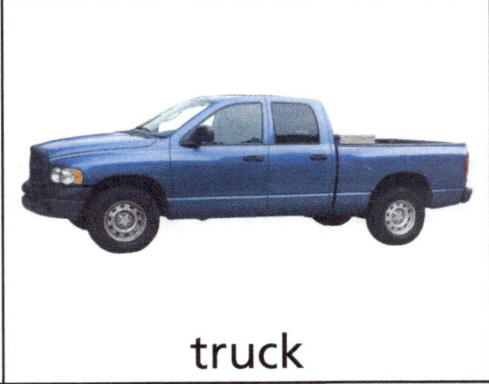 truck
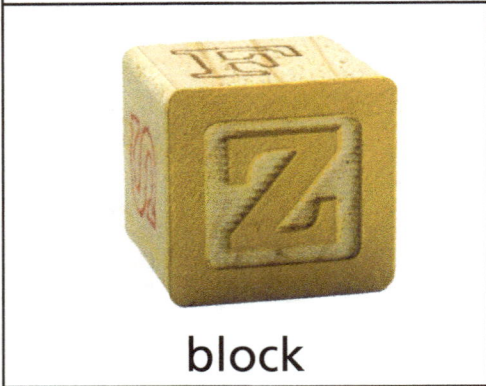 block	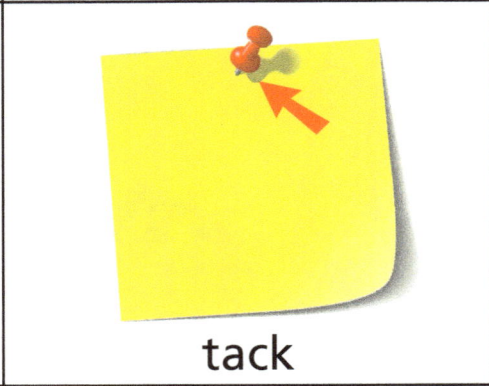 tack	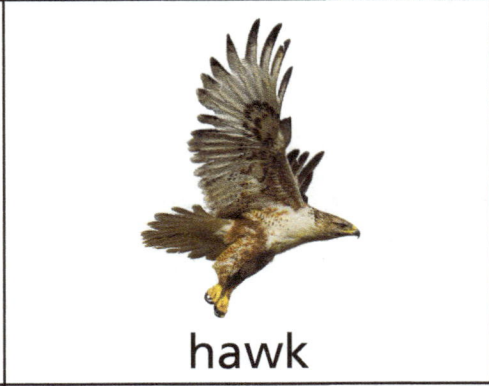 hawk
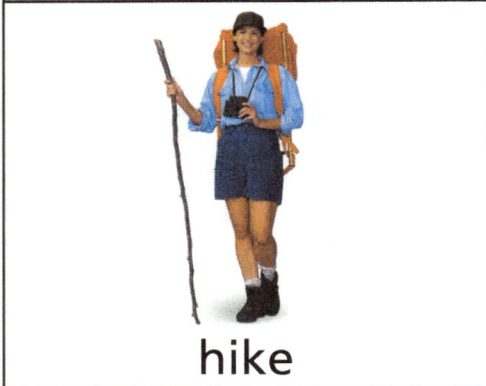 hike	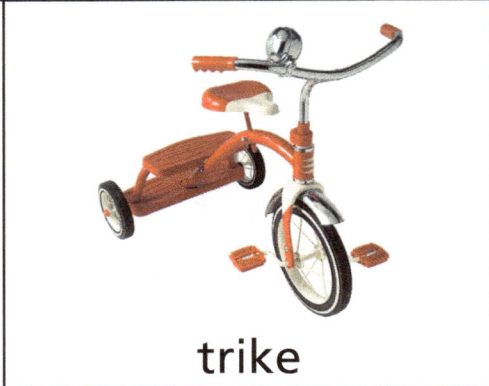 trike	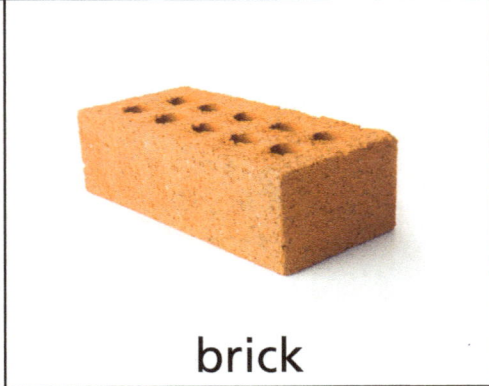 brick

Name _____

Helper Signature _____

Speech - Language Pathologist _____

Date _____

#BKCD-273 • Say & Do® Artic Reps • ©2015 Super Duper® Publications • www.superduperinc.com

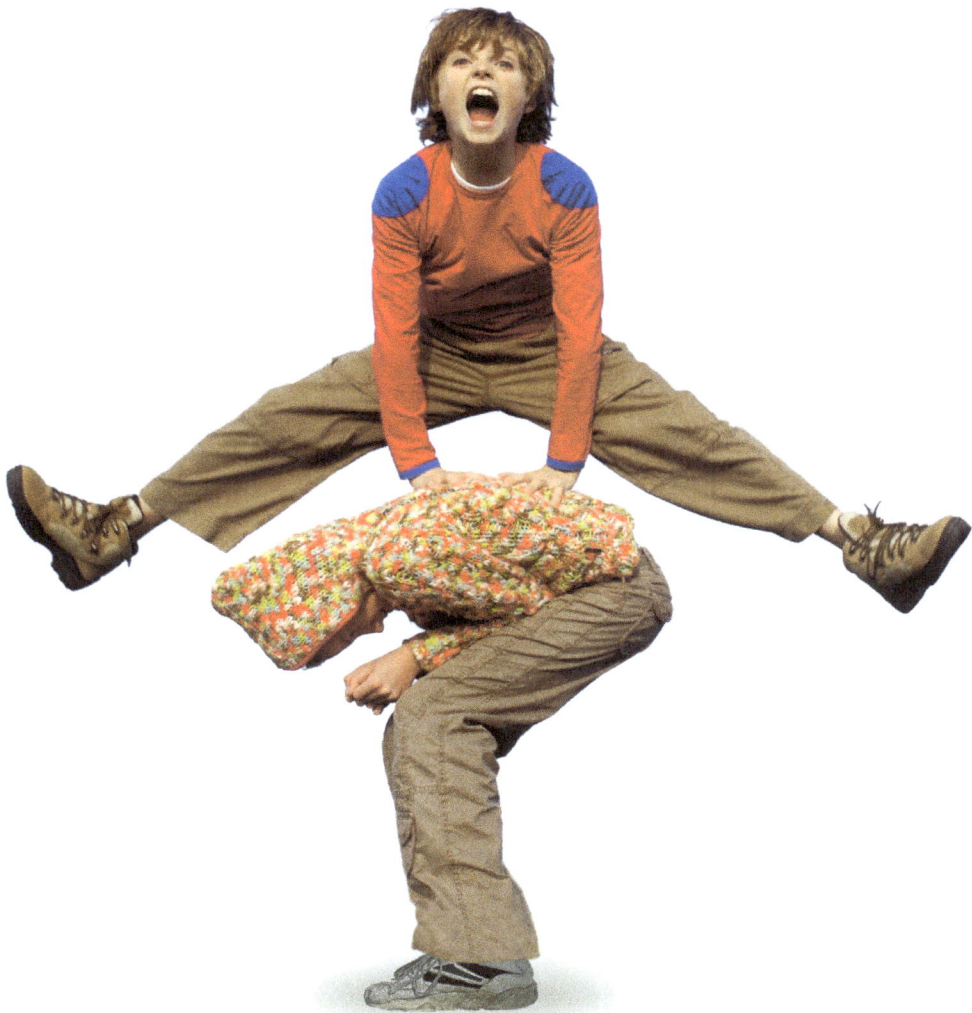

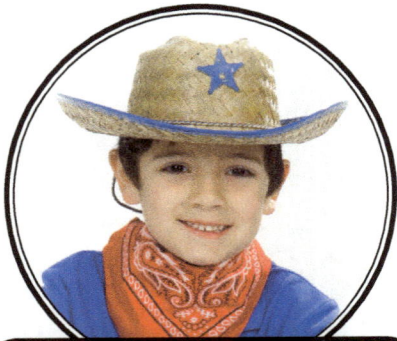

Larry

This is Larry. He laughed at all the things on this page.

1. Practice your sound by saying the words on this page. (Ex. lettuce, ladybug, etc.). Say the last word twice.

2. Practice saying **Larry** with each of the words. (Ex. Larry lettuce, Larry ladybug, etc.). Say the last word pair twice.

3. Practice saying **laughed at** in these words. (Ex. Larry laughed at lettuce, etc.). Say one of the sentences twice.

4. Practice saying **large** with these words. (Larry laughed at the large lettuce, etc.). Say one of the expanded sentences twice.

When you have finished this whole page you will have said your sound in 100 words! Good job!

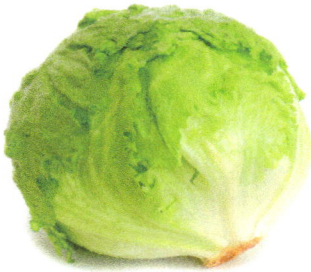 lettuce	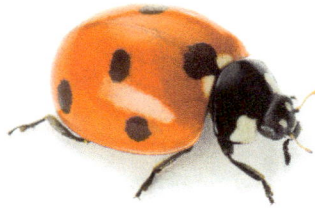 ladybug	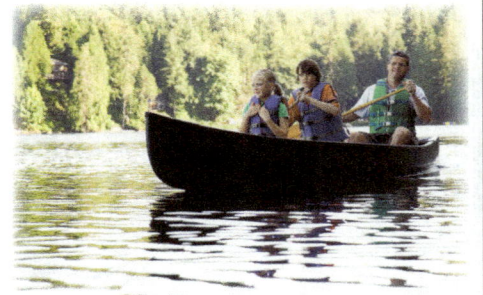 lake
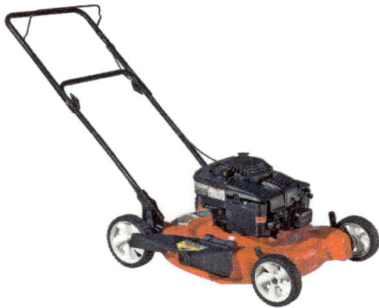 lawn mower	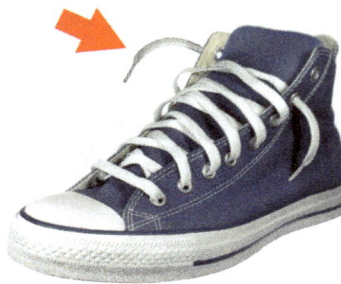 lace	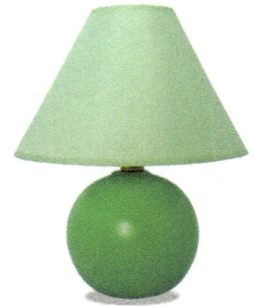 lamp
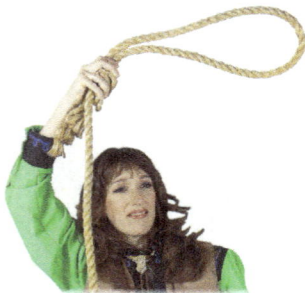 lasso	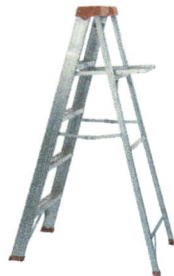 ladder	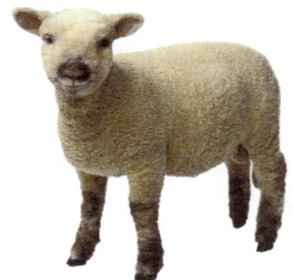 lamb

Name _____

Speech - Language Pathologist _____

Helper Signature _____

Date _____

#BKCD-273 • *Say & Do® Artic Reps* • ©2015 Super Duper® Publications • www.superduperinc.com

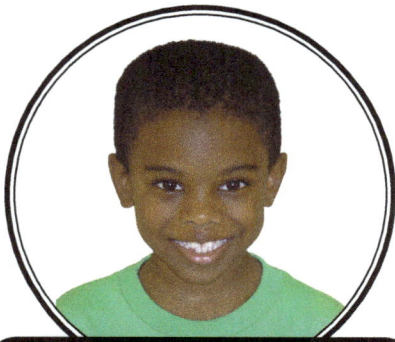

Lee

This is Lee. He left all the things on this page.

1. Practice your sound by saying the words on this page. (Ex. lemonade, lady, etc.). Say the last word twice.

2. Practice saying **Lee** with each of the words. (Ex. Lee lemonade, Lee lady, etc.). Say the last word pair twice.

3. Practice saying **left** with these words. (Ex. Lee left lemonade, etc.). Say one of the sentences twice.

4. Practice saying **leather** with these words. (Lee left leather lemonade, etc.). Say one of the expanded sentences twice.

When you have finished this whole page you will have said your sound in 100 words! Good job!

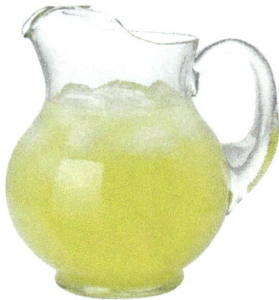	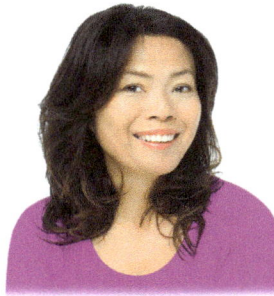	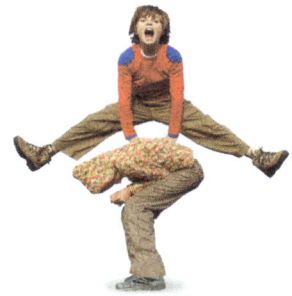
lemonade	lady	leapfrog
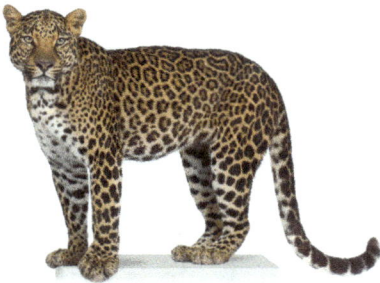	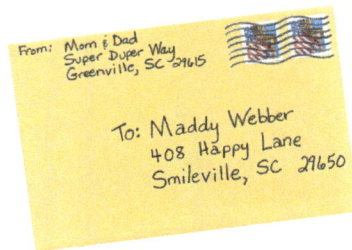	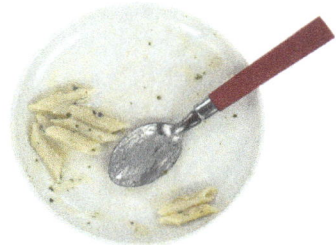
leopard	letter	leftovers
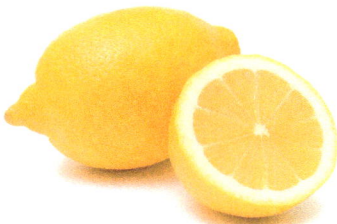	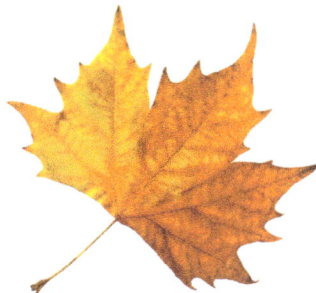	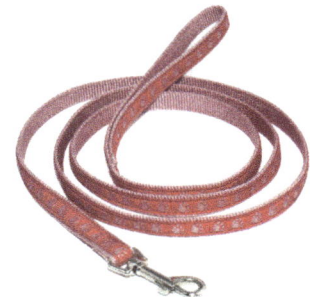
lemon	leaf	leash

Name _____

Helper Signature _____

Speech - Language Pathologist _____

Date _____

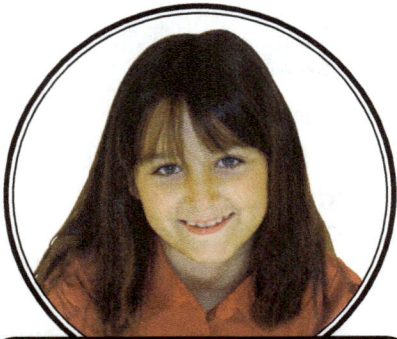

Lynn

This is Lynn. She likes all the things on this page.

L – Initial Position

1. Practice your sound by saying the words on this page. (Ex. limes, library, etc.). Say the last word twice.

2. Practice saying **Lynn** with each of the words. (Ex. Lynn limes, Lynn library, etc.). Say the last word pair twice.

3. Practice saying **likes** with these words. (Ex. Lynn likes limes, etc.). Say one of the sentences twice.

4. Practice saying **little** with these words. (Lynn likes little limes, etc.). Say one of the expanded sentences twice.

When you have finished this whole page you will have said your sound in 100 words! Good job!

limes	library	limo
lion	licorice	lizard
lifeguard	lighthouse	lid

Name _____

Helper Signature _____

Speech - Language Pathologist _____

Date _____

#BKCD-273 • *Say & Do® Artic Reps* • ©2015 Super Duper® Publications • www.superduperinc.com

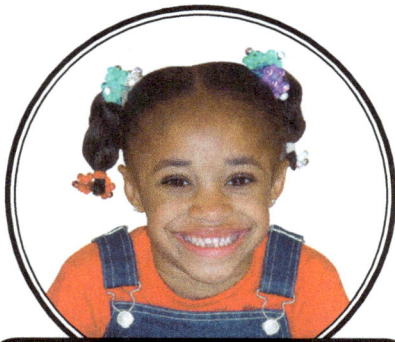

Lois

This is Lois. She lost all the things on this page.

L – Initial Position

1. Practice your sound by saying the words on this page. (Ex. loaf, lobster, etc.). Say the last word twice.

2. Practice saying **Lois** with each of the words. (Ex. Lois loaf, Lois lobster, etc.). Say the last word pair twice.

3. Practice saying **lost** with these words. (Ex. Lois lost a loaf, etc.). Say one of the sentences twice.

4. Practice saying **long** with these words. (Lois lost a long loaf etc.). Say one of the expanded sentences twice.

When you have finished this whole page you will have said your sound in 100 words! Good job!

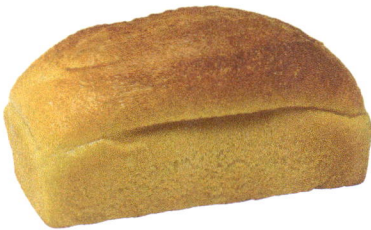 loaf	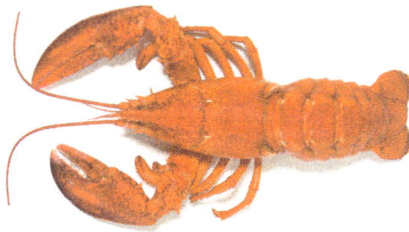 lobster	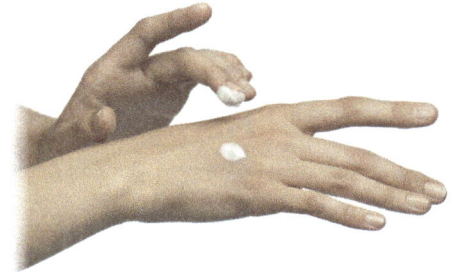 lotion
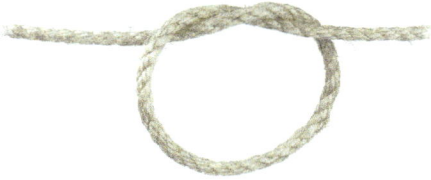 loop	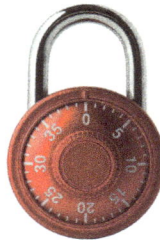 lock	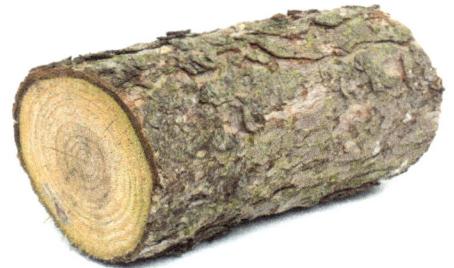 log
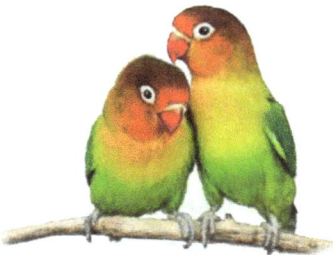 lovebirds	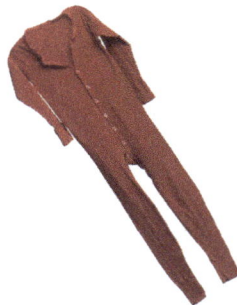 long johns	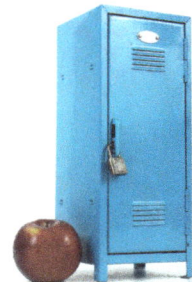 locker

Name _____

Helper Signature _____

Speech - Language Pathologist _____

Date _____

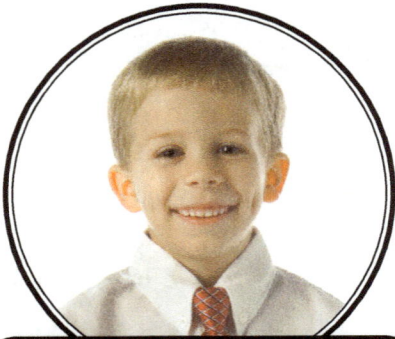

Luke

This is Luke. He looks at all the things on this page.

L – Initial Position

1. Practice your sound by saying the words on this page. (Ex. lung, lumber, etc.). Say the last word twice.

2. Practice saying **Luke** with each of the words. (Ex. Luke lung, Luke lumber, etc.). Say the last word pair twice.

3. Practice saying **looks at** with these words. (Ex. Luke looks at a lung, etc.). Say one of the sentences twice.

4. Practice saying **loud** with these words. (Luke looks at a loud lung, etc.). Say one of the expanded sentences twice.

   When you have finished this whole page you will have said your sound in 100 words! Good job!

lung	lumber	lump
luggage	lunch	lunch meat
lunchroom	lumberjack	lawn

Name

Speech - Language Pathologist

Helper Signature

Date

#BKCD-273 • *Say & Do® Artic Reps* • ©2015 Super Duper® Publications • www.superduperinc.com

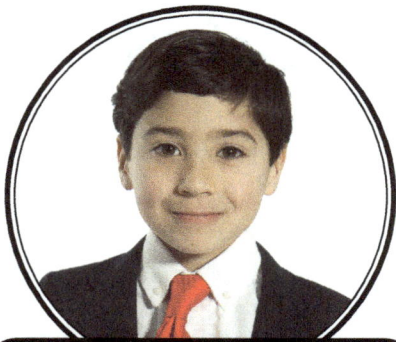

Allen

This is Allen. He was feeling all the things on this page.

1. Practice your sound by saying the words on this page. (Ex. balloons, wallet, etc.). Say the last word twice.

2. Practice saying **Allen** with each of the words. (Ex. Allen balloons, Allen wallet, etc.). Say the last word pair twice.

3. Practice saying **was feeling** with these words. (Ex. Allen was feeling the balloons, etc.). Say one of the sentences twice.

4. Practice saying **jolly** with these words. (Allen was feeling the jolly balloons, etc.). Say one of the expanded sentences twice.

When you have finished this whole page you will have said your sound in 100 words! Good job!

balloons	wallet	dollar
umbrella	telephone	walnut
telescope	dandelion	envelope

Name _____

Helper Signature _____

Speech - Language Pathologist _____

Date _____

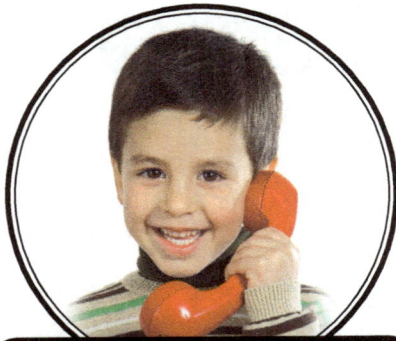

Billy

This is Billy. He was selling all the things on this page.

1. Practice your sound by saying the words on this page. (Ex. television, melon, etc.). Say the last word twice.

2. Practice saying **Billy** with each of the words. (Ex. Billy television, Billy melon, etc.). Say the last word pair twice.

3. Practice saying **was selling** with these words. (Ex. Billy was selling a television, etc.). Say one of the sentences twice.

4. Practice saying **ugly** with these words. (Billy was selling an ugly television, etc.). Say one of the expanded sentences twice.

When you have finished this whole page you will have said your sound in 100 words! Good job!

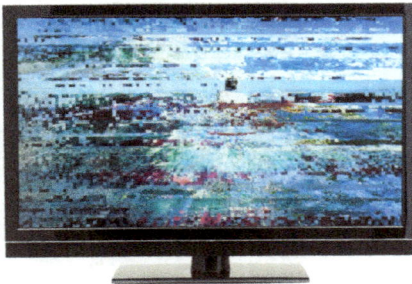 television	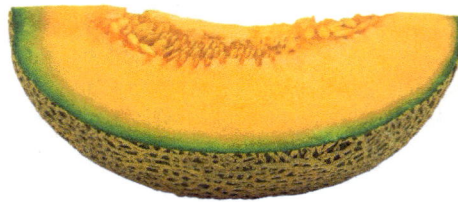 melon	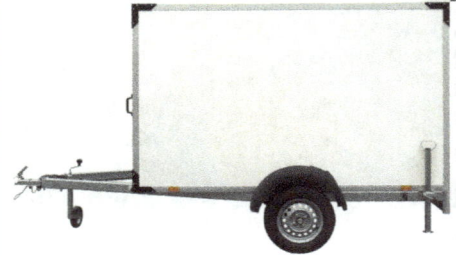 trailer
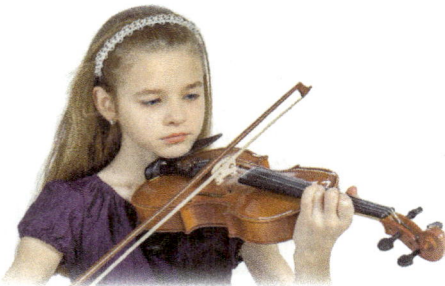 violin	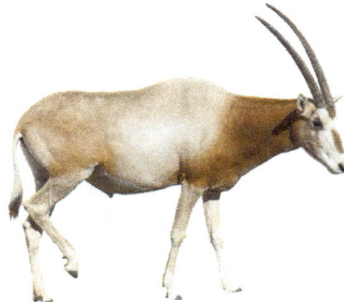 antelope	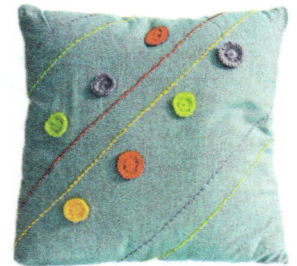 pillow
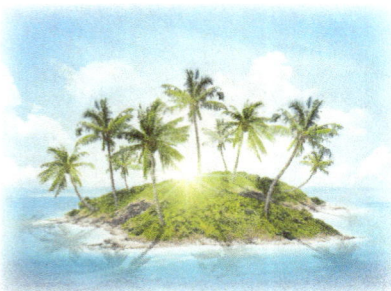 island	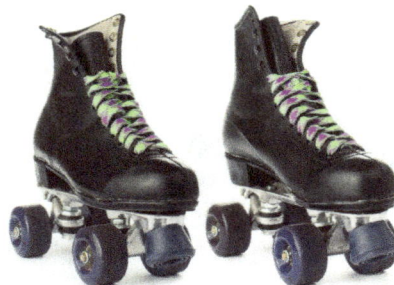 roller skates	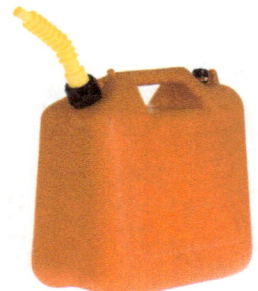 gasoline

Name

Helper Signature

Speech - Language Pathologist

Date

#BKCD-273 • *Say & Do® Artic Reps* • ©2015 Super Duper® Publications • www.superduperinc.com

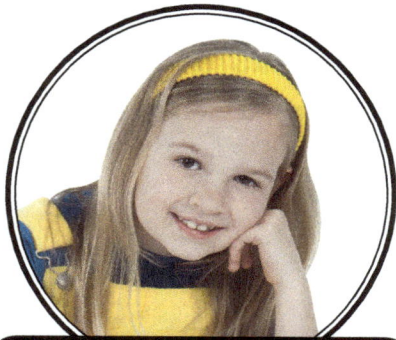

Julie

This is Julie. She was following all the things on this page.

L – Medial Position

1. Practice your sound by saying the words on this page. (Ex. elephant, ambulance, etc.). Say the last word twice.

2. Practice saying **Julie** with each of the words. (Ex. Julie elephant, Julie ambulance, etc.). Say the last word pair twice.

3. Practice saying **was following** with these words. (Ex. Julie was following an elephant, etc.). Say one of the sentences twice.

4. Practice saying **silly** with these words. (Julie was following a silly elephant, etc.). Say one of the expanded sentences twice.

When you have finished this whole page you will have said your sound in 100 words! Good job!

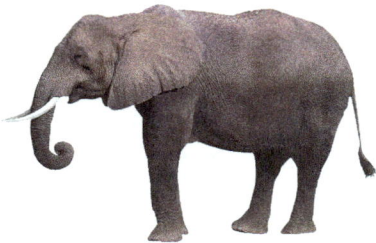

elephant

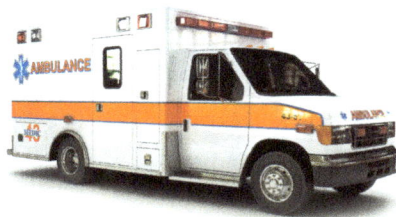

ambulance

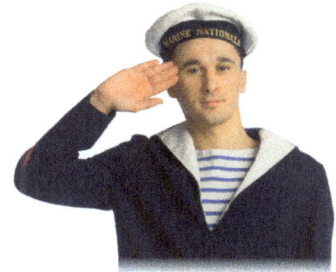

sailor

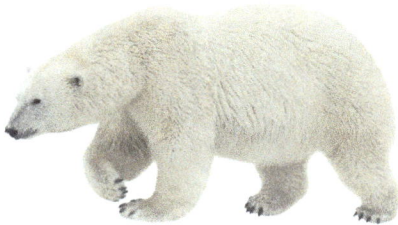

polar bear

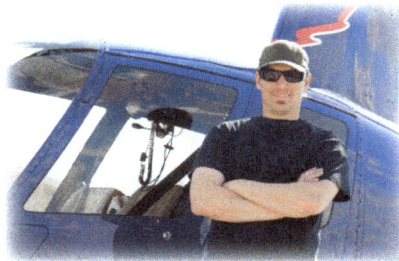

pilot

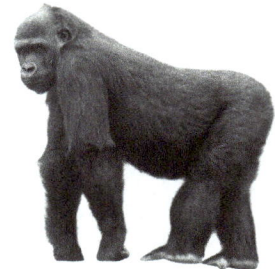

gorilla

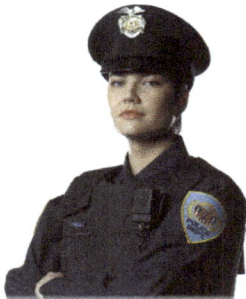

police

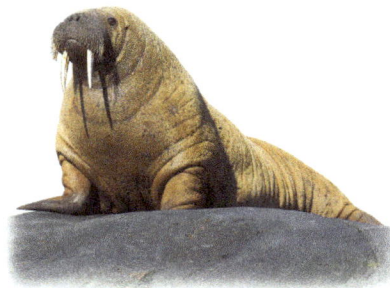

walrus

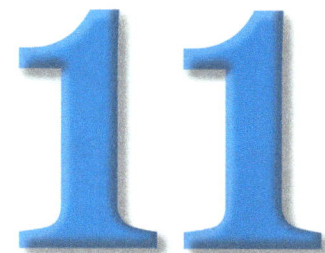

eleven

Name

Helper Signature

Speech - Language Pathologist

Date

L – Medial Position

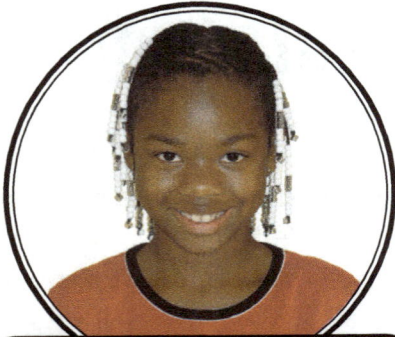

Keely

1. Practice your sound by saying the words on this page. (Ex. jelly, celery, etc.). Say the last word twice.

2. Practice saying **Keely** with each of the words. (Ex. Keely jelly, Keely celery, etc.). Say the last word pair twice.

3. Practice saying **was swallowing** with these words. (Ex. Keely was swallowing jelly, etc.). Say one of the sentences twice.

4. Practice saying **delicious** with these words. (Keely was swallowing delicious jelly, etc.). Say one of the expanded sentences twice.

This is Keely. She was swallowing all the things on this page.

When you have finished this whole page you will have said your sound in 100 words! Good job!

jelly	celery	chili
gelatin	broccoli	chocolate
watermelon	bologna	salad

Name _____

Helper Signature _____

Speech - Language Pathologist _____

Date _____

#BKCD-273 • *Say & Do® Artic Reps* • ©2015 Super Duper® Publications • www.superduperinc.com

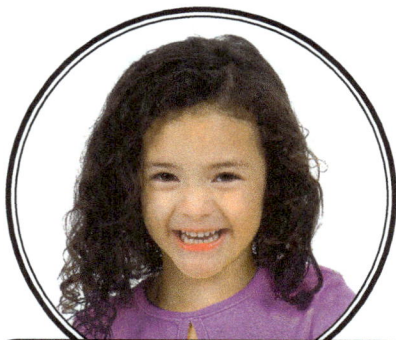

Val

This is Val. She fell on all the things on this page.

1. Practice your sound by saying the words on this page. (Ex. sandpile, snowball, etc.). Say the last word twice.

2. Practice saying **Val** with each of the words. (Ex. Val sandpile, Val snowball, etc.). Say the last word pair twice.

3. Practice saying **fell on** with these words. (Ex. Val fell on a sandpile, etc.). Say one of the sentences twice.

4. Practice saying **small** with these words. (Val fell on a small sandpile, etc.). Say one of the expanded sentences twice.

When you have finished this whole page you will have said your sound in 100 words! Good job!

sandpile	snowball	anthill
pail	ball	toadstool
shovel	doll	football

Name _____

Helper Signature _____

Speech - Language Pathologist _____

Date _____

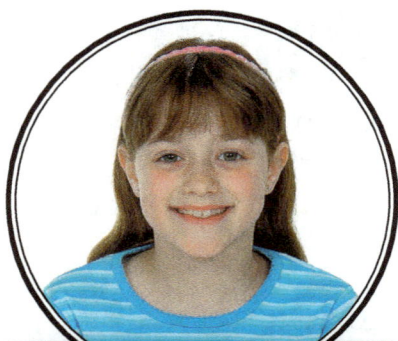

Jill

This is Jill. She can feel all the things on this page.

1. Practice your sound by saying the words on this page. (Ex. towel, beach ball, etc.). Say the last word twice.

2. Practice saying **Jill** with each of the words. (Ex. Jill towel, Jill beach ball, etc.). Say the last word pair twice.

3. Practice saying **can feel** with these words. (Ex. Jill can feel a towel, etc.). Say one of the phrases twice.

4. Practice saying **tall** with these words. (Jill can feel a tall towel, etc.). Say one of the sentences twice.

   When you have finished this whole page you will have said your sound in 100 words! Good job!

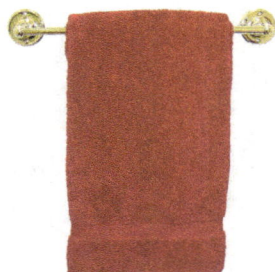 **towel**	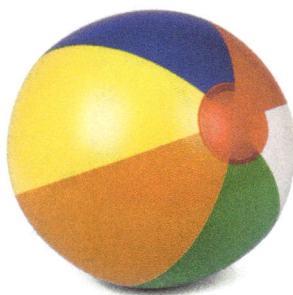 **beach ball**	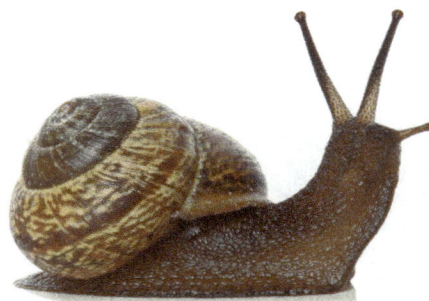 **snail**
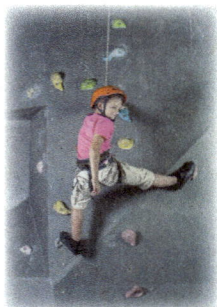 **wall**	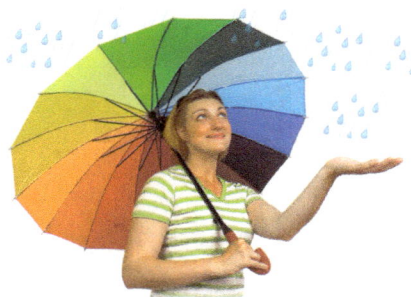 **rainfall**	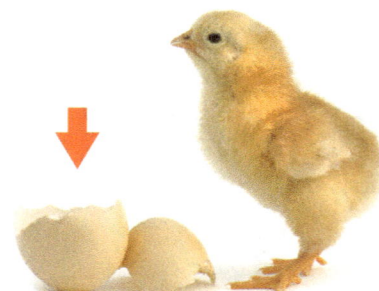 **eggshell**
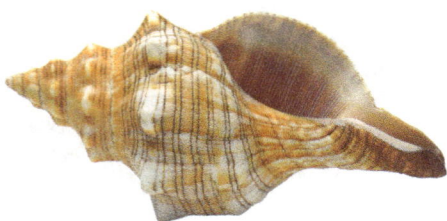 **seashell**	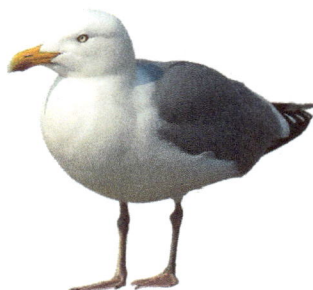 **seagull**	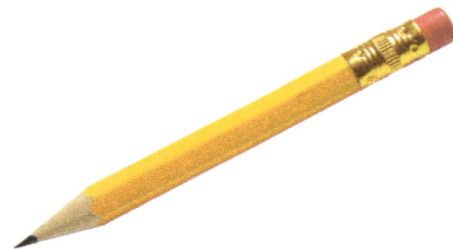 **pencil**

Name _____

Speech - Language Pathologist _____

Helper Signature _____

Date _____

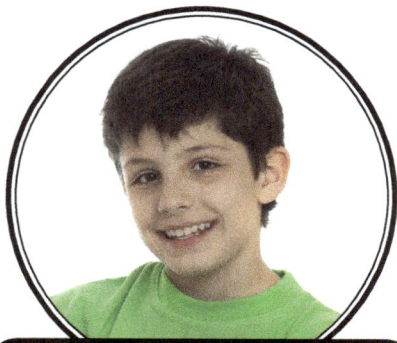

Paul

This is Paul. He can smell all the things on this page.

1. Practice your sound by saying the words on this page. (Ex. owl, whale, etc.). Say the last word twice.

2. Practice saying **Paul** with each of the words. (Ex. Paul owl, Paul whale, etc.). Say the last word pair twice.

3. Practice saying **can smell** with these words. (Ex. Paul can smell an owl, etc.). Say one of the sentences twice.

4. Practice saying **cool** with these words. (Paul can smell a cool owl, etc.). Say one of the expanded sentences twice.

When you have finished this whole page you will have said your sound in 100 words! Good job!

owl	whale	waffle
well	coal	wheel
casserole	oatmeal	pinwheel

Name _____

Speech - Language Pathologist _____

Helper Signature _____

Date _____

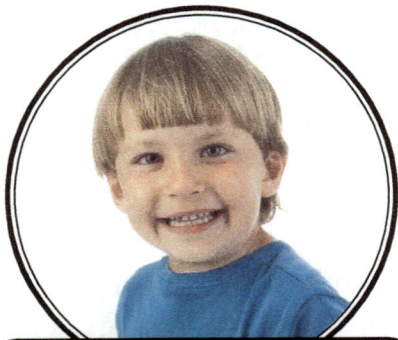

Kyle

This is Kyle. He can sell all the things on this page.

L – Final Position

1. Practice your sound by saying the words on this page. (Ex. shawl, parasol, etc.). Say the last word twice.

2. Practice saying **Kyle** with each of the words. (Ex. Kyle shawl, Kyle parasol, etc.). Say the last word pair twice.

3. Practice saying **can sell** with these words. (Ex. Kyle can sell a shawl, etc.). Say one of the sentences twice.

4. Practice saying **beautiful** with these words. (Kyle can sell a beautiful shawl, etc.). Say one of the expanded sentences twice.

When you have finished this whole page you will have said your sound in 100 words! Good job!

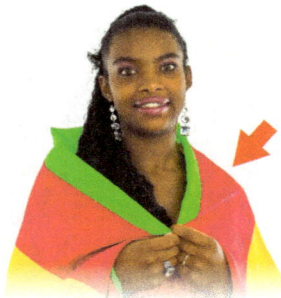 shawl	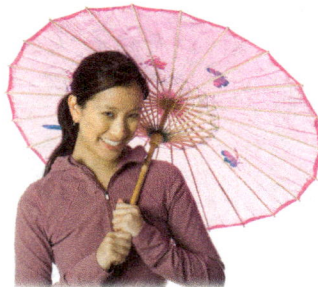 parasol	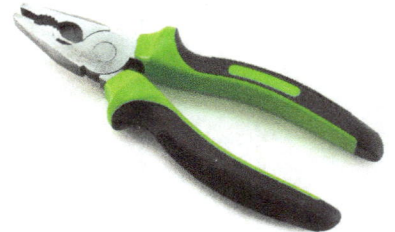 tool
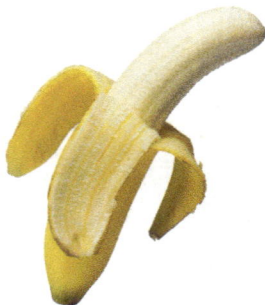 peel	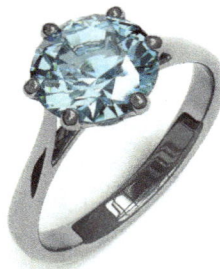 jewel	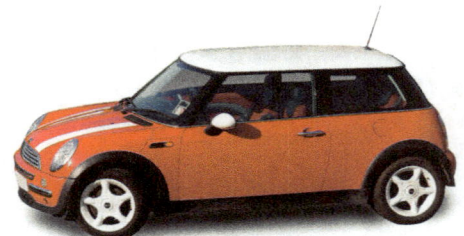 automobile
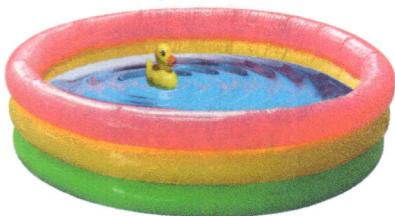 pool	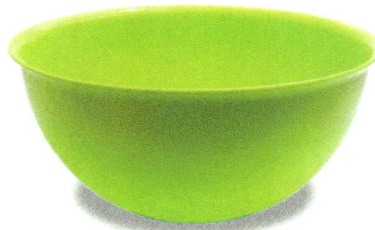 bowl	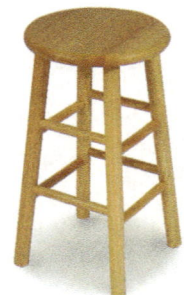 stool

Name _____

Helper Signature _____

Speech - Language Pathologist _____

Date _____

#BKCD-273 • *Say & Do® Artic Reps* • ©2015 Super Duper® Publications • www.superduperinc.com

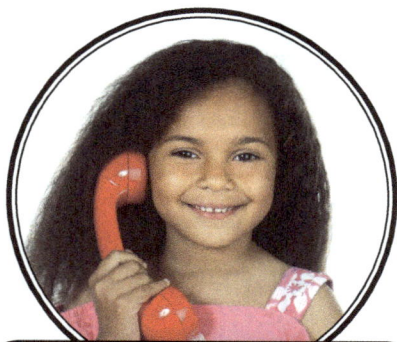

Blanche

This is Blanche. She blabbed about all the things on this page.

1. Practice your sound by saying the words on this page. (Ex. blue jeans, blouse, etc.). Say the last word twice.

2. Practice saying **Blanche** with each of the words. (Ex. Blanche blue jeans, Blanche blouse, etc.). Say the last word pair twice.

3. Practice saying **blabbed about** with these words. (Ex. Blanche blabbed about blue jeans, etc.). Say one of the sentences twice.

4. Practice saying **blue** with these words. (Blanche blabbed about blue blue jeans, etc.). Say one of the expanded sentences twice.

When you have finished this whole page you will have said your sound in 100 words! Good job!

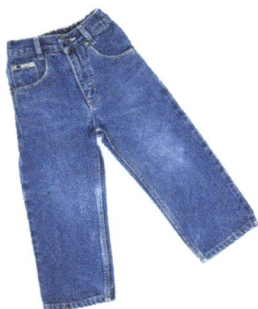 blue jeans	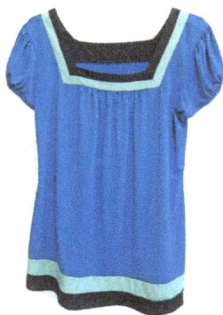 blouse	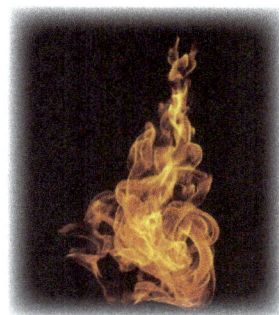 blaze
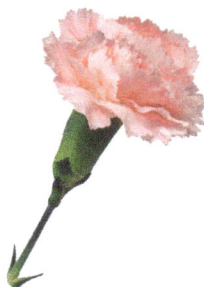 blossom	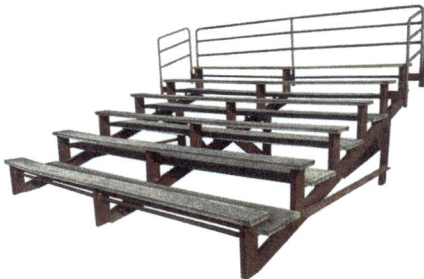 bleachers	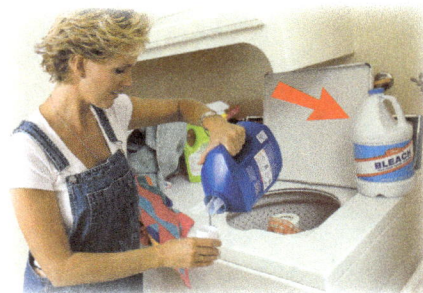 bleach
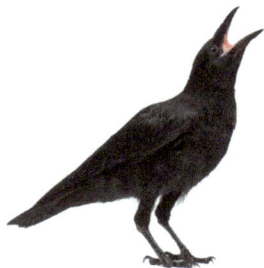 blackbird	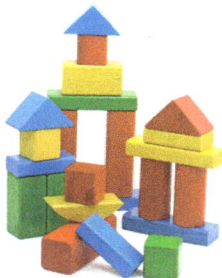 blocks	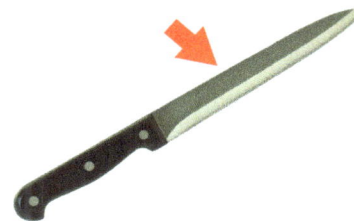 blade

Name _____

Helper Signature _____

Speech - Language Pathologist _____

Date _____

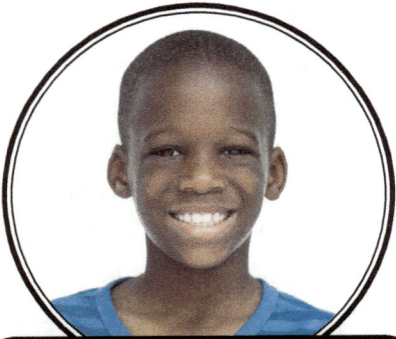

Blake

This is Blake. He blamed all the things on this page.

1. Practice your sound by saying the words on this page. (Ex. blanket, blue whale, etc.). Say the last word twice.

2. Practice saying **Blake** with each of the words. (Ex. Blake blanket, Blake blue whale, etc.). Say the last word pair twice.

3. Practice saying **blamed** with these words. (Ex. Blake blamed a blanket, etc.). Say one of the sentences twice.

4. Practice saying **blemished** with these words. (Blake blamed a blemished blanket, etc.). Say one of the expanded sentences twice.

When you have finished this whole page you will have said your sound in 100 words! Good job!

blanket	blue whale	blindfold
blimp	blonde	blow
blue jay	blender	sibling

Name _____

Helper Signature _____

Speech - Language Pathologist _____

Date _____

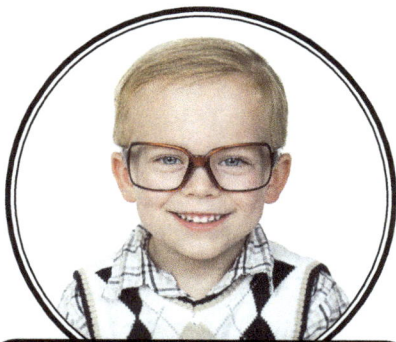

Floyd

This is Floyd. He fled from all the things on this page.

FL – Blend

1. Practice your sound by saying the words on this page. (Ex. dragonfly, flippers, etc.). Say the last word twice.

2. Practice saying **Floyd** with each of the words. (Ex. Floyd dragonfly, Floyd flippers, etc.). Say the last word pair twice.

3. Practice saying **fled from** with these words. (Ex. Floyd fled from a dragonfly, etc.). Say one of the sentences twice.

4. Practice saying **flat** with these words. (Floyd fled from a flat dragonfly, etc.). Say one of the expanded sentences twice.

When you have finished this whole page you will have said your sound in 100 words! Good job!

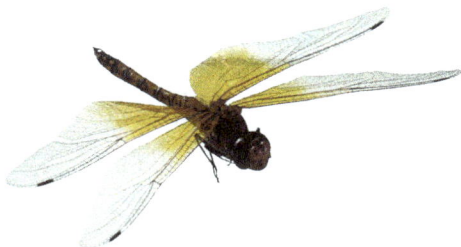 dragonfly	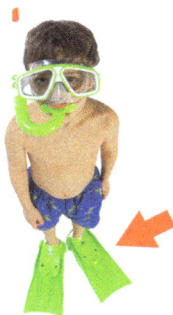 flippers	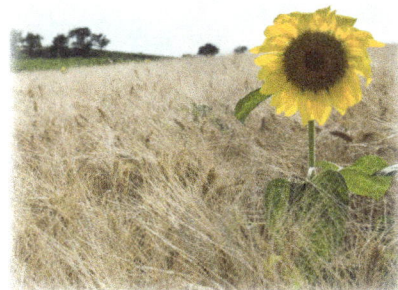 sunflower
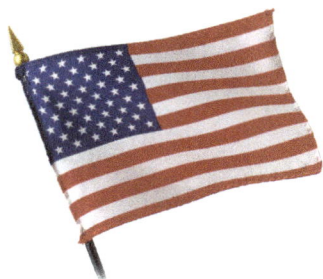 flag	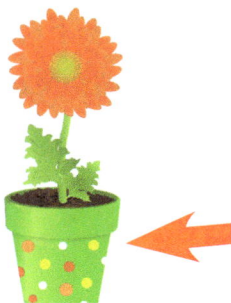 flowerpot	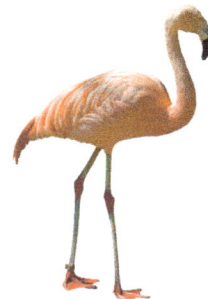 flamingo
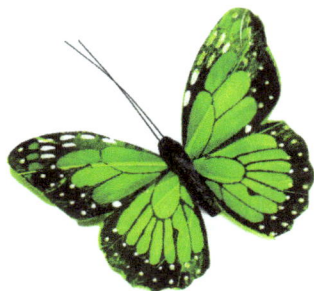 butterfly	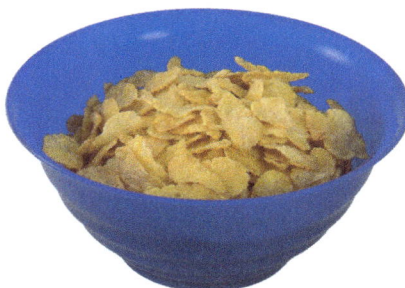 cornflakes	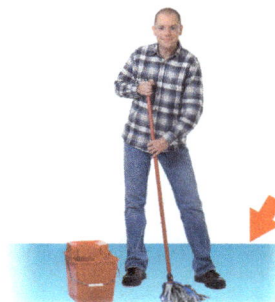 floor

Name _____

Helper Signature _____

Speech - Language Pathologist _____

Date _____

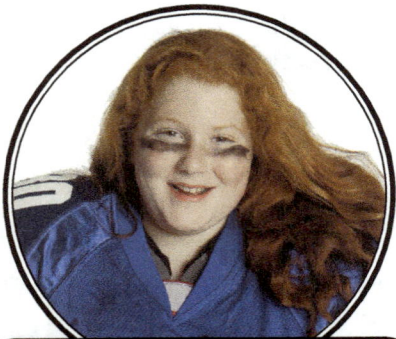

FL – Blend

Flo

This is Flo. She flipped all the things on this page.

1. Practice your sound by saying the words on this page. (Ex. flame, snowflake, etc.). Say the last word twice.

2. Practice saying **Flo** with each of the words. (Ex. Flo flame, Flo snowflake, etc.). Say the last word pair twice.

3. Practice saying **flipped** with these words. (Ex. Flo flipped the flame, etc.). Say one of the sentences twice.

4. Practice saying **floppy** with these words. (Flo flipped a floppy flame, etc.). Say one of the expanded sentences twice.

When you have finished this whole page you will have said your sound in 100 words! Good job!

flame	snowflake	flute
flapjacks	flea	flower
flash cards	fly	float

Name _____

Speech - Language Pathologist _____

Helper Signature _____

Date _____

#BKCD-273 • *Say & Do® Artic Reps* • ©2015 Super Duper® Publications • www.superduperinc.com

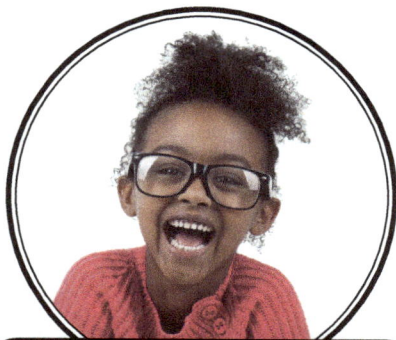

Gloria

This is Gloria. She glazed all the things on this page.

GL – Blend

1. Practice your sound by saying the words on this page. (Ex. boxing glove, globe, etc.). Say the last word twice.

2. Practice saying **Gloria** with each of the words. (Ex. Gloria boxing glove, Gloria globe, etc.). Say the last word pair twice.

3. Practice saying **glazed** with these words. (Ex. Gloria glazed a boxing glove, etc.). Say one of the sentences twice.

4. Practice saying **glowing** with these words. (Gloria glazed a glowing boxing glove, etc.). Say one of the expanded sentences twice.

When you have finished this whole page you will have said your sound in 100 words! Good job!

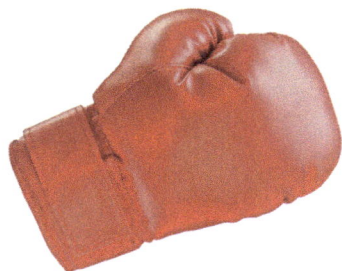 boxing glove	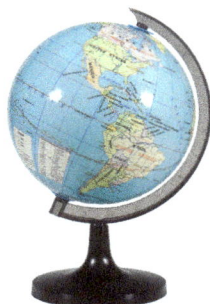 globe	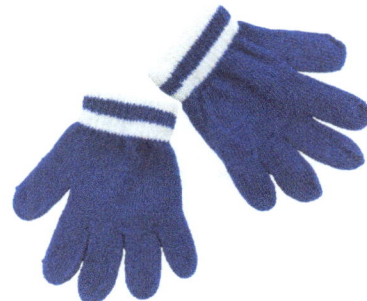 gloves
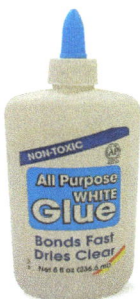 glue	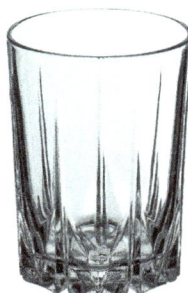 glass	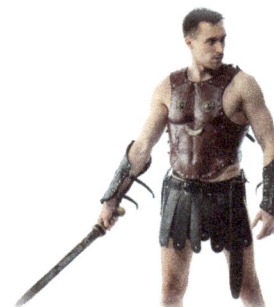 gladiator
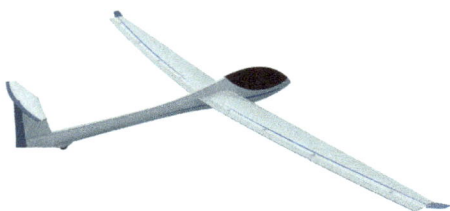 glider	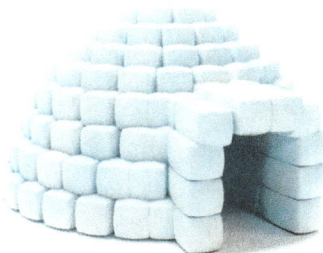 igloo	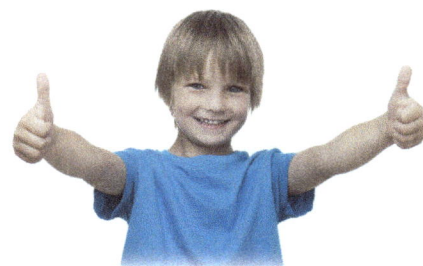 glad

Name _____

Helper Signature _____

Speech - Language Pathologist _____

Date _____

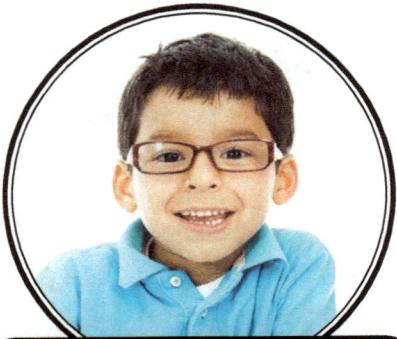

Glenn

This is Glenn. He glanced at all the things on this page.

GL – Blend

1. Practice your sound by saying the words on this page. (Ex. glitter, glasses, etc.). Say the last word twice.

2. Practice saying **Glenn** with each of the words. (Ex. Glenn glitter, Glenn glasses, etc.). Say the last word pair twice.

3. Practice saying **glanced at** with these words. (Ex. Glenn glanced at glitter, etc.). Say one of the sentences twice.

4. Practice saying **glamorous** with these words. (Glenn glanced at glamorous glitter, etc.). Say one of the expanded sentences twice.

When you have finished this whole page you will have said your sound in 100 words! Good job!

glitter	glasses	juggler
hourglass	lip gloss	glowing pumpkin
glacier	glazed doughnut	piglet

Name _____

Speech - Language Pathologist _____

Helper Signature _____

Date _____

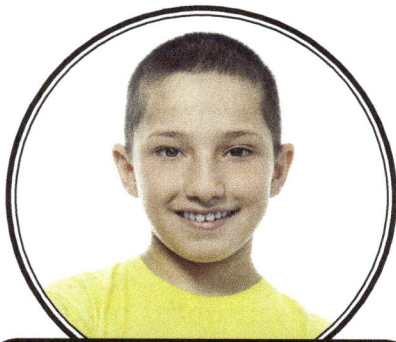

Clint

This is Clint. He climbed on all the things on this page.

KL – Blend

1. Practice your sound by saying the words on this page. (Ex. clay, cliff, etc.). Say the last word twice.

2. Practice saying **Clint** with each of the words. (Ex. Clint clay, Clint cliff, etc.). Say the last word pair twice.

3. Practice saying **climbed on** with these words. (Ex. Clint climbed on clay, etc.). Say one of the sentences twice.

4. Practice saying **clean** with these words. (Clint climbed on clean clay, etc.). Say one of the expanded sentences twice.

When you have finished this whole page you will have said your sound in 100 words! Good job!

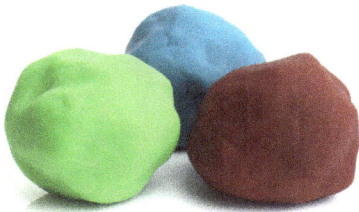 clay	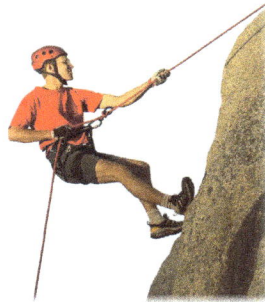 cliff	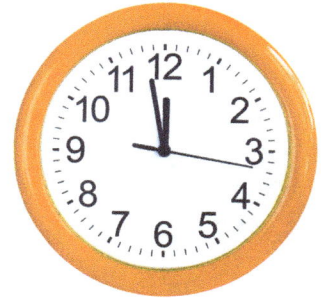 clock
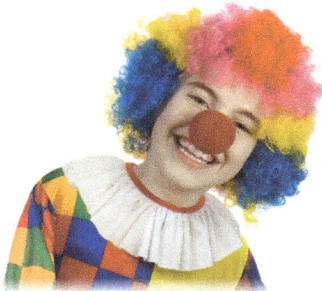 clown	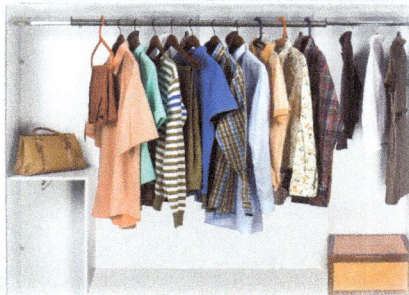 closet	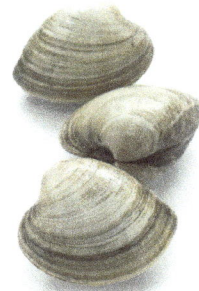 clams
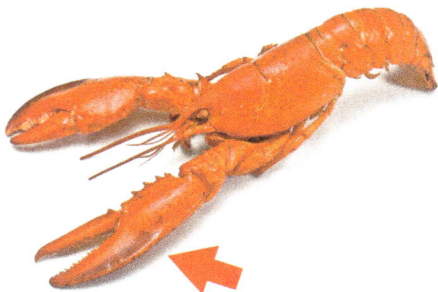 claw	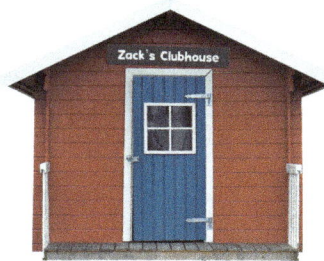 clubhouse	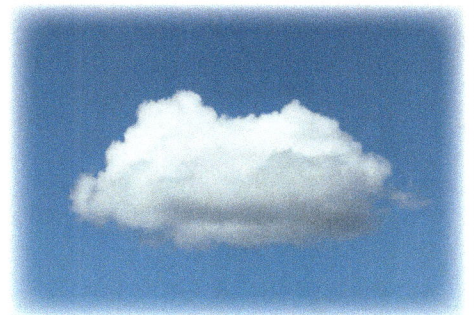 cloud

Name _____

Helper Signature _____

Speech - Language Pathologist _____

Date _____

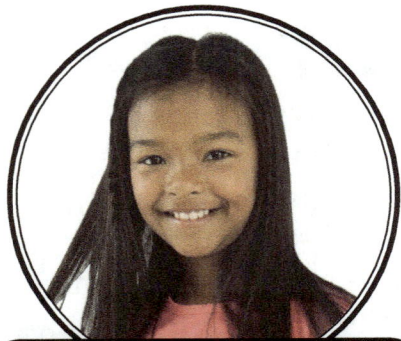

Clarissa

This is Clarissa. She clapped about all the things on this page.

1. Practice your sound by saying the words on this page. (Ex. clasp, class, etc.). Say the last word twice.

2. Practice saying **Clarissa** with each of the words. (Ex. Clarissa clasp, Clarissa class, etc.). Say the last word pair twice.

3. Practice saying **clapped about** with these words. (Ex.Clarissa clapped about a clasp, etc.). Say one of the sentences twice.

4. Practice saying **clever** with these words. (Claire clapped about a clever clasp, etc.). Say one of the expanded sentences twice.

When you have finished this whole page you will have said your sound in 100 words! Good job!

clasp	class	clue
clothes	clothespin	cluster
clearance	classroom	club sandwich

Name _____

Helper Signature _____

Speech - Language Pathologist _____

Date _____

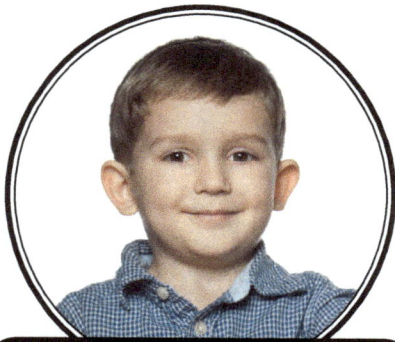

Pluto

This is Pluto. He plants all the things on this page.

PL – Blend

1. Practice your sound by saying the words on this page. (Ex. place mat, plum, etc.). Say the last word twice.
2. Practice saying **Pluto** with each of the words. (Ex. Pluto place mat, Pluto plum, etc.). Say the last word pair twice.
3. Practice saying **plants** with these words. (Ex. Pluto plants a place mat, etc.). Say one of the sentences twice.
4. Practice saying **plain** with these words. (Pluto plants a plain place mat, etc.). Say one of the expanded sentences twice.

When you have finished this whole page you will have said your sound in 100 words! Good job!

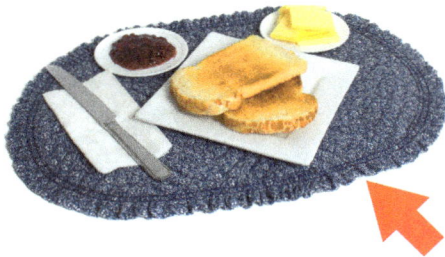 place mat	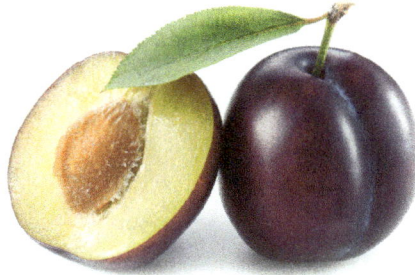 plum	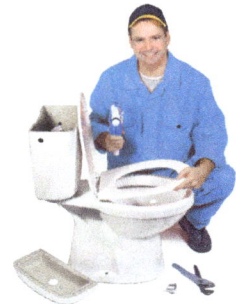 plumber
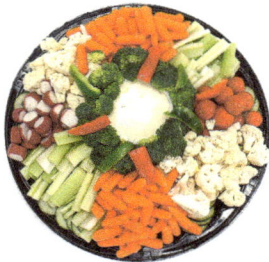 platter	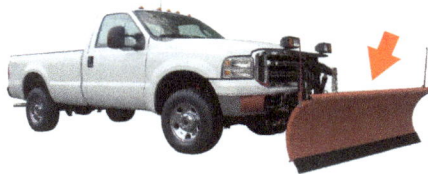 plow	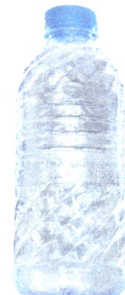 plastic
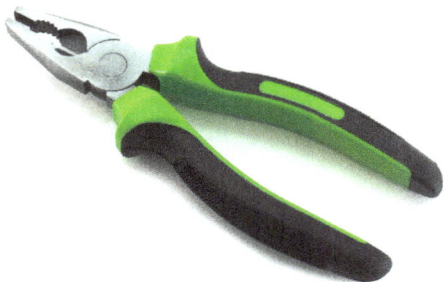 pliers	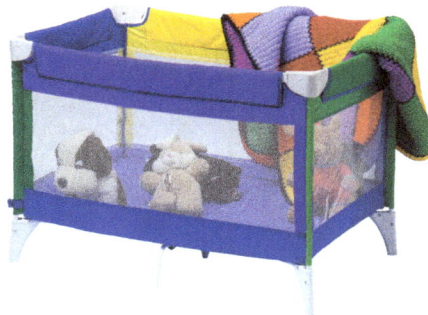 playpen	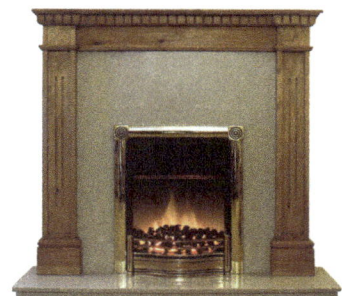 fireplace

Name _____

Speech - Language Pathologist _____

Helper Signature _____

Date _____

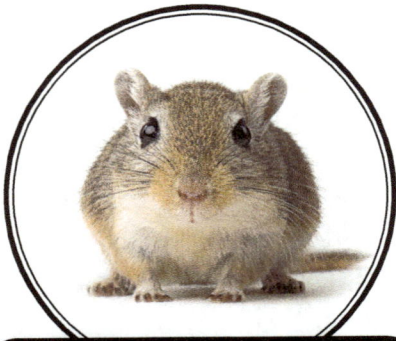

Plink

PL – Blend

1. Practice your sound by saying the words on this page. (Ex. plant, airplane, etc.). Say the last word twice.

2. Practice saying **Plink** with each of the words. (Ex. Plink plant, Plink airplane, etc.). Say the last word pair twice.

3. Practice saying **played** with these words. (Ex. Plink played with the plant, etc.). Say one of the sentences twice.

4. Practice saying **plump** with these words. (Plink played with a plump plant, etc.). Say one of the expanded sentences twice.

This is Plink. She played with all the things on this page.

When you have finished this whole page you will have said your sound in 100 words! Good job!

plant	airplane	platypus
playhouse	planet	plate
eggplant	playing cards	plug

Name _____

Helper Signature _____

Speech - Language Pathologist _____

Date _____

#BKCD-273 • Say & Do® Artic Reps • ©2015 Super Duper® Publications • www.superduperinc.com

R

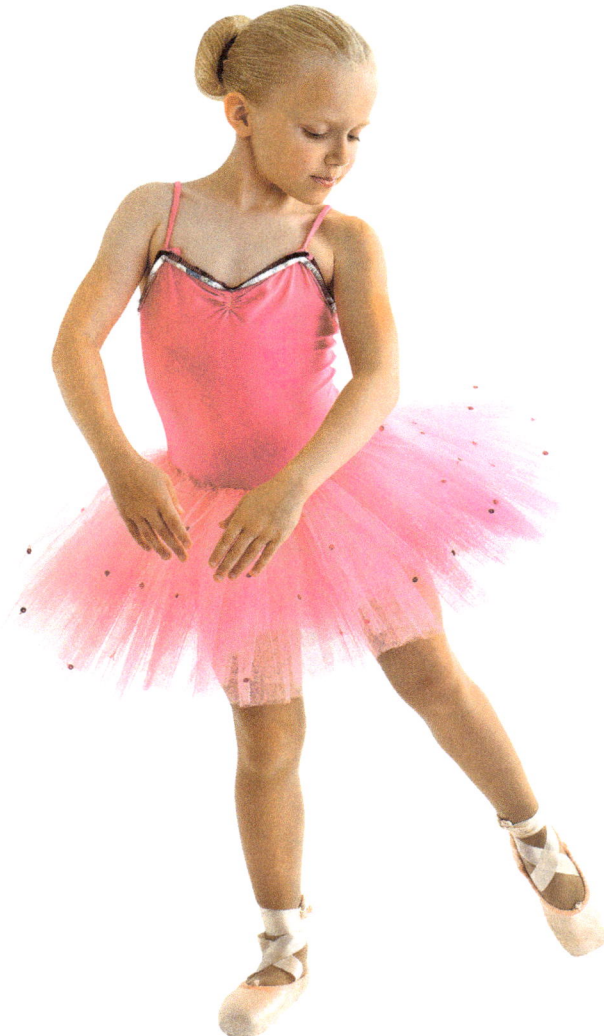

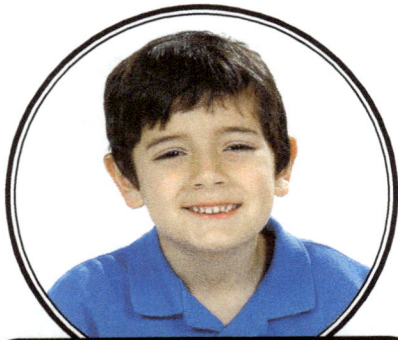

Ray

This is Ray. He wrapped all the things on this page.

1. Practice your sound by saying the words on this page. (Ex. rake, raisins, etc.). Say the last word twice.

2. Practice saying **Ray** with each of the words. (Ex. Ray rake, Ray raisins, etc.). Say the last word pair twice.

3. Practice saying **wrapped** with these words. (Ex. Ray wrapped the rake, etc.). Say one of the sentences twice.

4. Practice saying **ragged** with these words. (Ray wrapped a ragged rake, etc.). Say one of the expanded sentences twice.

When you have finished this whole page you will have said your sound in 100 words! Good job!

rake	raisins	rainbow
rag	racket	rabbit
radio	raccoon	rat

Name

Speech - Language Pathologist

Helper Signature

Date

#BKCD-273 • *Say & Do*® Artic Reps • ©2015 Super Duper® Publications • www.superduperinc.com

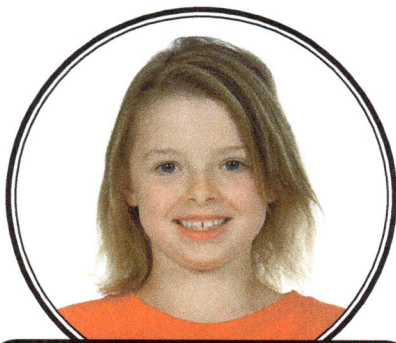

Reba

This is Reba. She rescued all the things on this page.

1. Practice your sound by saying the words on this page. (Ex. reptile, wren, etc.). Say the last word twice.

2. Practice saying **Reba** with each of the words. (Ex. Reba reptile, Reba wren, etc.). Say the last word pair twice.

3. Practice saying **rescued** with these words. (Ex. Reba rescued a reptile, etc.). Say one of the sentences twice.

4. Practice saying **red** with these words. (Reba rescued a red reptile, etc.). Say one of the expanded sentences twice.

When you have finished this whole page you will have said your sound in 100 words! Good job!

reptile	wren	remote
wrench	wreath	rectangle
wreck	relative	radio

Name _____

Helper Signature _____

Speech - Language Pathologist _____

Date _____

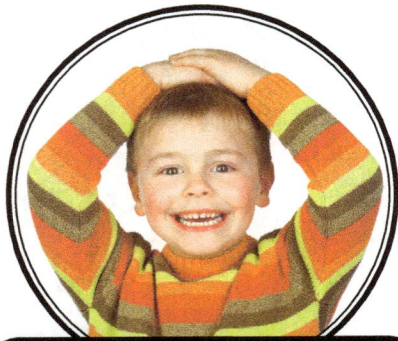

Rick

This is Rick. He rinsed all the things on this page.

1. Practice your sound by saying the words on this page. (Ex. rhino, rings, etc.). Say the last word twice.

2. Practice saying **Rick** with each of the words. (Ex. Rick rhino, Rick rings, etc.). Say the last word pair twice.

3. Practice saying **rinsed** with these words. (Ex. Rick rinsed the rhino, etc.). Say one of the sentences twice.

4. Practice saying **right** with these words. (Rick rinsed the right rhino, etc.). Say one of the expanded sentences twice.

When you have finished this whole page you will have said your sound in 100 words! Good job!

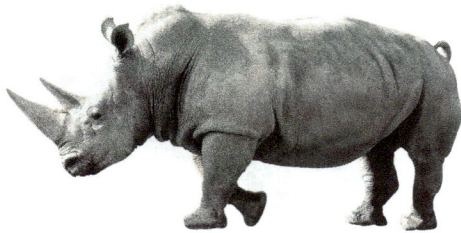 rhino	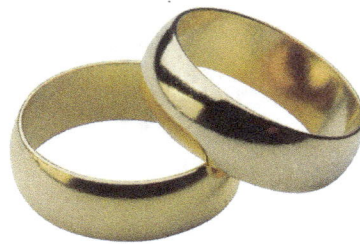 rings	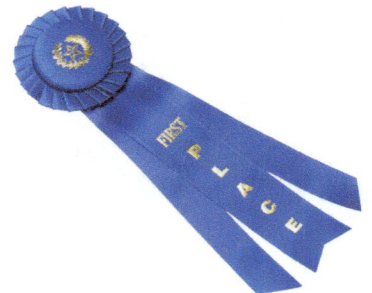 ribbon
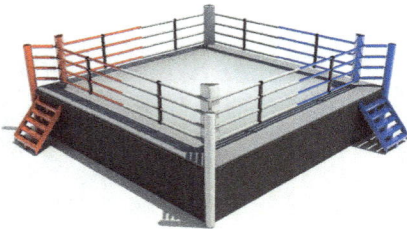 ring	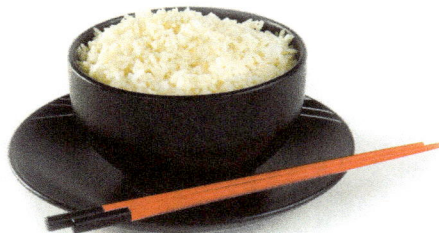 rice	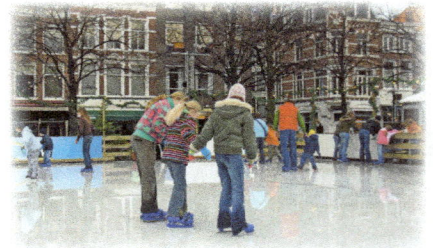 rink
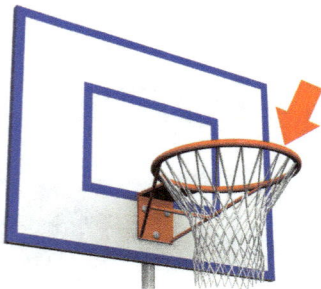 rim	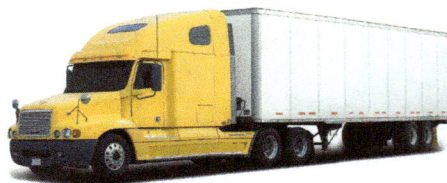 rig	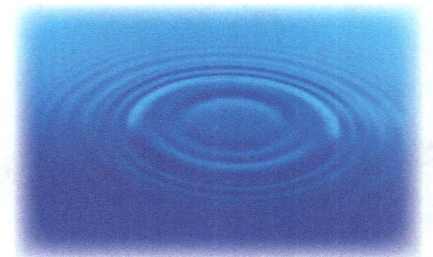 ripple

Name _____

Helper Signature _____

Speech - Language Pathologist _____

Date _____

#BKCD-273 • *Say & Do® Artic Reps* • ©2015 Super Duper® Publications • www.superduperinc.com

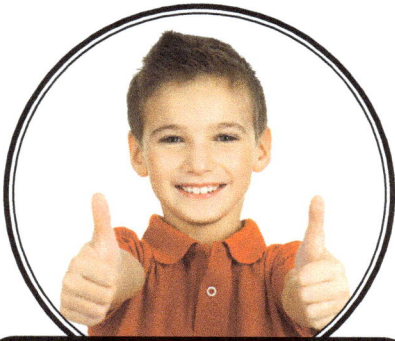

Ron

This is Ron. He rode all the things on this page.

R – Prevocalic

1. Practice your sound by saying the words on this page. (Ex. rod, rope, etc.). Say the last word twice.

2. Practice saying **Ron** with each of the words. (Ex. Ron rod, Ron rope, etc.). Say the last word pair twice.

3. Practice saying **rode** with these words. (Ex. Ron rode a fishing rod, etc.). Say one of the sentences twice.

4. Practice saying **round** with these words. (Ron rode a round fishing rod, etc.). Say one of the expanded sentences twice.

When you have finished this whole page you will have said your sound in 100 words! Good job!

fishing rod	rope	rose
roast beef	rock	robot
robin	rocket	rowboat

Name _____

Helper Signature _____

Speech - Language Pathologist _____

Date _____

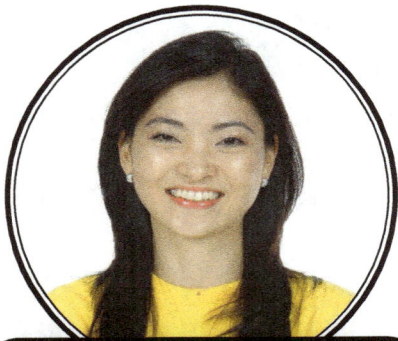

Ruby

This is Ruby. She rubs all the things on this page.

1. Practice your sound by saying the words on this page. (Ex. root, rubber bands, etc.). Say the last word twice.

2. Practice saying **Ruby** with each of the words. (Ex. Ruby root, Ruby rubber bands, etc.). Say the last word pair twice.

3. Practice saying **rubs** with these words. (Ex. Ruby rubs a root, etc.). Say one of the phrases twice.

4. Practice saying **rusty** with these words. (Ruby rubs a rusty root, etc.). Say one of the sentences twice.

When you have finished this whole page you will have said your sound in 100 words! Good job!

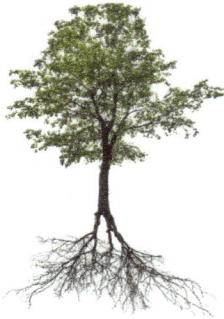 roots	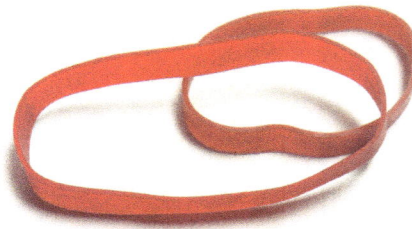 rubber bands	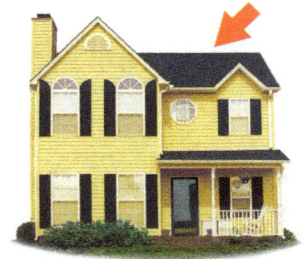 roof
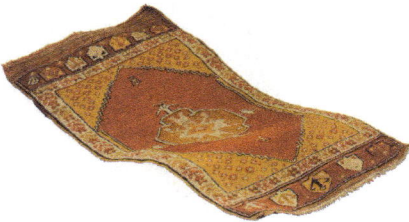 rug	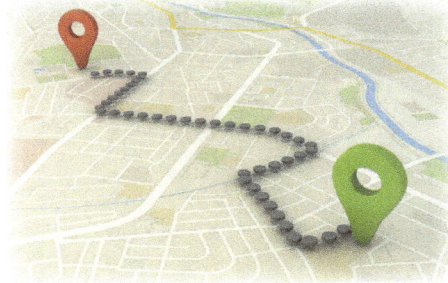 route	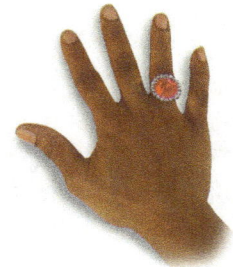 ruby
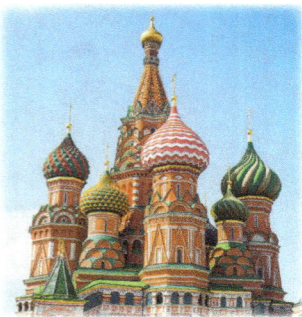 Russia	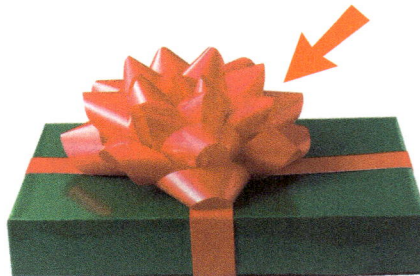 ribbon	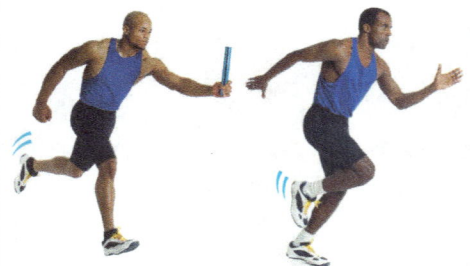 race

Name _____

Helper Signature _____

Speech - Language Pathologist _____

Date _____

#BKCD-273 • *Say & Do® Artic Reps* • ©2015 Super Duper® Publications • www.superduperinc.com

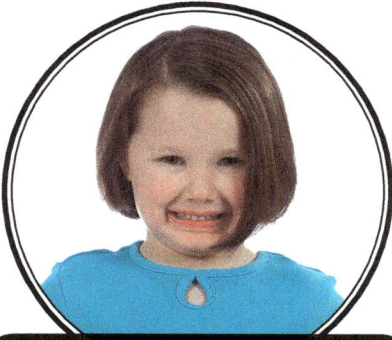

R – Vocalic AR

1. Practice your sound by saying the words on this page. (Ex. car, starfish, etc.). Say the last word twice.
2. Practice saying **Margaret** with each of the words. (Ex. Margaret car, Margaret starfish, etc.). Say the last word pair twice.
3. Practice saying **parked beside** with these words. (Ex. Margaret parked beside a car, etc.). Say one of the sentences twice.
4. Practice saying **bizarre** with these words. (Margaret parked beside a bizarre car, etc.). Say one of the expanded sentences twice.

When you have finished this whole page you will have said your sound in 100 words! Good job!

Margaret

This is Margaret. She parked beside all the things on this page.

car	starfish	scar
apartment	party	armadillo
garden	arm	barn

Name _____

Helper Signature _____

Speech - Language Pathologist _____

Date _____

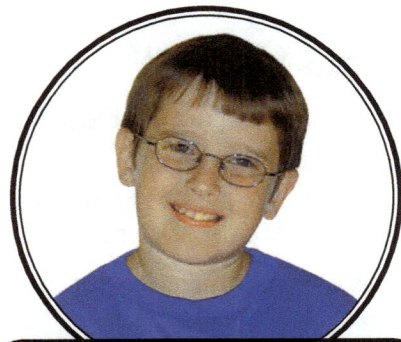

R – Vocalic AR

Carson

This is Carson. He was borrowing all the things on this page.

1. Practice your sound by saying the words on this page. (Ex. jar, guitar, etc.). Say the last word twice.
2. Practice saying **Carson** with each of the words. (Ex. Carson jar, Carson guitar, etc.). Say the last word pair twice.
3. Practice saying **was borrowing** with these words. (Ex. Carson was borrowing a jar, etc.). Say one of the sentences twice.
4. Practice saying **large** with these words. (Carson was borrowing a large jar, etc.). Say one of the expanded sentences twice.

When you have finished this whole page you will have said your sound in 100 words! Good job!

jar	guitar	heart
yarn	harp	star
marbles	target	cards

Name _____

Helper Signature _____

Speech - Language Pathologist _____

Date _____

#BKCD-273 • *Say & Do® Artic Reps* • ©2015 Super Duper® Publications • www.superduperinc.com

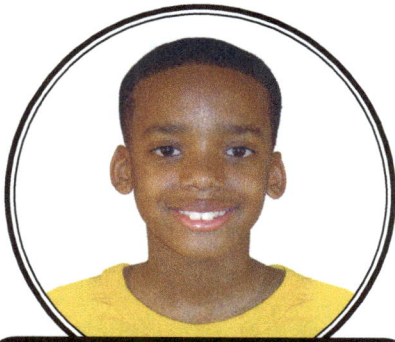

Peter

This is Peter. He will twirl all the things on this page.

1. Practice your sound by saying the words on this page. (Ex. battery, beaver, etc.). Say the last word twice.

2. Practice saying **Peter** with each of the words. (Ex. Peter battery, Peter beaver, etc.). Say the last word pair twice.

3. Practice saying **will observe** with these words. (Ex. Peter will observe the battery, etc.). Say one of the sentences twice.

4. Practice saying **super** with these words. (Peter will observe a super battery, etc.). Say one of the expanded sentences twice.

When you have finished this whole page you will have said your sound in 100 words! Good job!

battery	beaver	otters
computer	winner	teacher
dancer	giraffe	ladder

Name _____

Helper Signature _____

Speech - Language Pathologist _____

Date _____

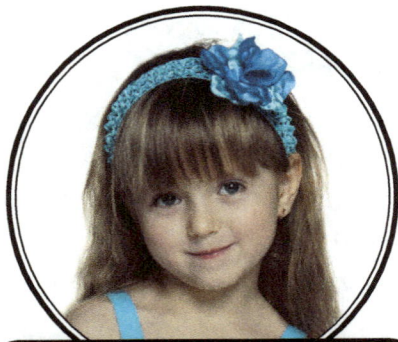

Heather

1. Practice your sound by saying the words on this page. (Ex. water, overalls, etc.). Say the last word twice.

2. Practice saying **Heather** with each of the words. (Ex. Heather water, Heather overalls, etc.). Say the last word pair twice.

3. Practice saying **will deliver** with these words. (Ex. Heather will deliver water, etc.). Say one of the sentences twice.

4. Practice saying **dirty** with these words. (Heather will deliver dirty water, etc.). Say one of the expanded sentences twice.

This is Heather. She will deliver all the things on this page.

When you have finished this whole page you will have said your sound in 100 words! Good job!

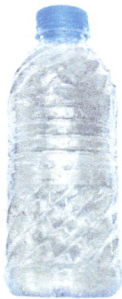 water	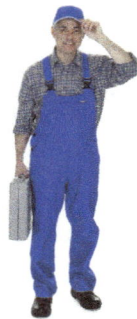 overalls	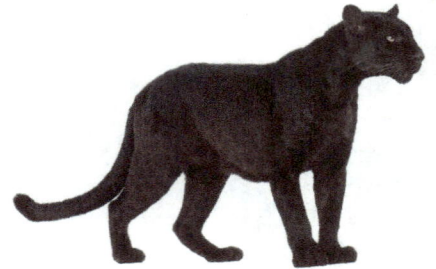 panther
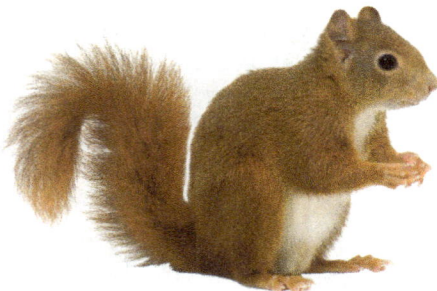 squirrel	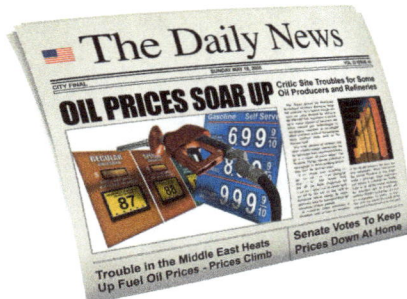 newspaper	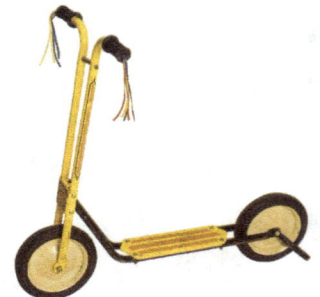 scooter
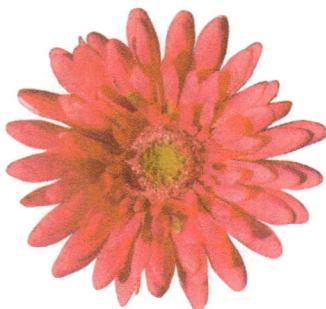 flower	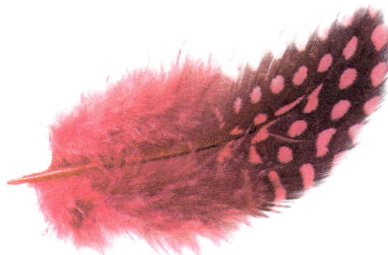 feather	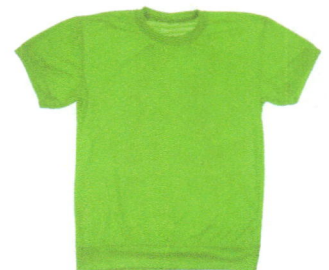 shirt

Name

Helper Signature

Speech - Language Pathologist

Date

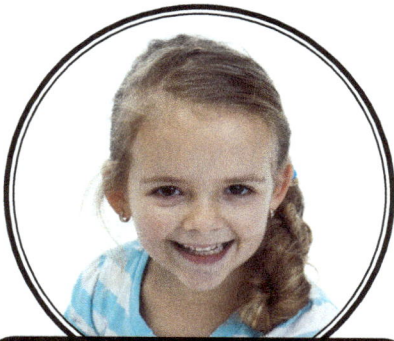

Lorie

This is Lorie. She ignores all the things on this page.

R – Vocalic OR

1. Practice your sound by saying the words on this page. (Ex. dinosaurs, oranges, etc.). Say the last word twice.
2. Practice saying **Lorie** with each of the words. (Ex. Lorie dinosaurs, Lorie oranges, etc.). Say the last word pair twice.
3. Practice saying **ignores** with these words. (Ex. Lorie ignores dinosaurs, etc.). Say one of the sentences twice.
4. Practice saying **four** with these words. (Lorie ignores four dinosaurs, etc.). Say one of the expanded sentences twice.

When you have finished this whole page you will have said your sound in 100 words! Good job!

dinosaurs	oranges	apple cores
orchids	scorpions	sports
forks	stories	horses

Name _____

Speech - Language Pathologist _____

Helper Signature _____

Date _____

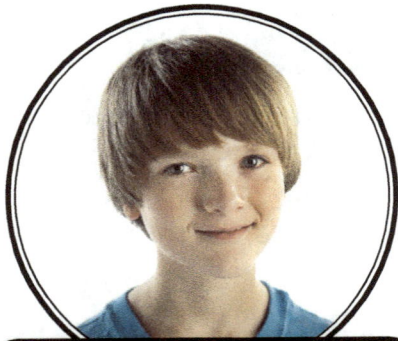

Corbin

This is Corbin. He adored all the things on this page.

R – Vocalic OR

1. Practice your sound by saying the words on this page. (Ex. doorbell, floor, etc.). Say the last word twice.

2. Practice saying **Corbin** with each of the words. (Ex. Corbin doorbell, Corbin floor, etc.). Say the last word pair twice.

3. Practice saying **adored** with these words. (Ex. Corbin adored a doorbell, etc.). Say one of the sentences twice.

4. Practice saying **boring** with these words. (Corbin adored a boring doorbell, etc.). Say one of the expanded sentences twice.

When you have finished this whole page you will have said your sound in 100 words! Good job!

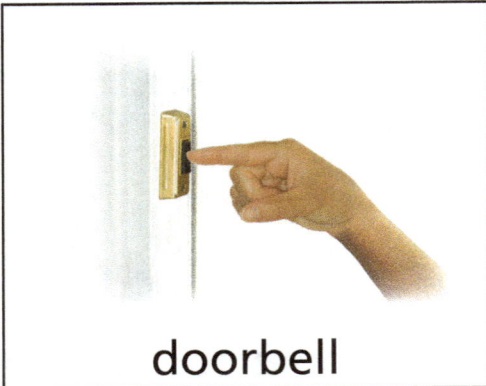 doorbell	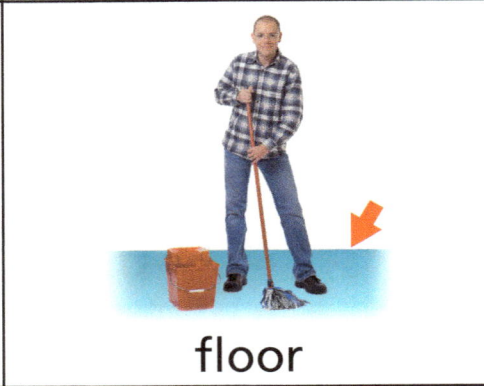 floor	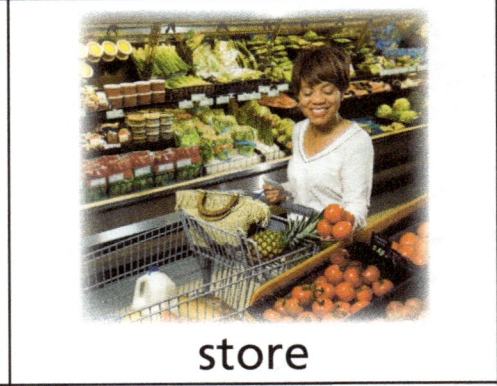 store
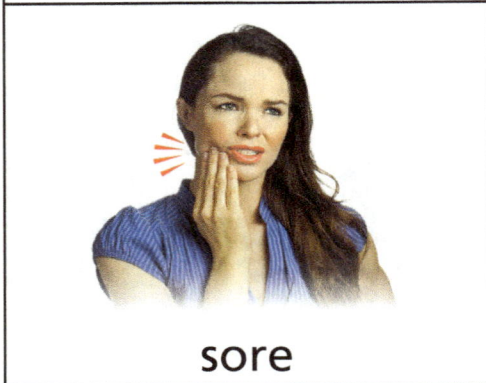 sore	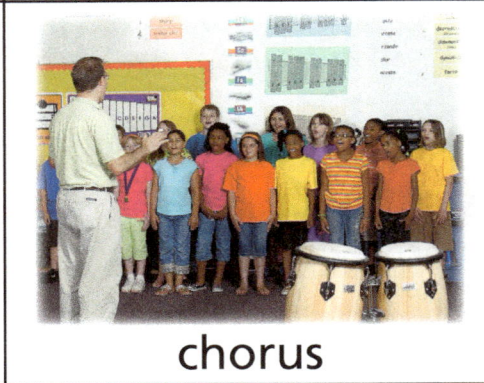 chorus	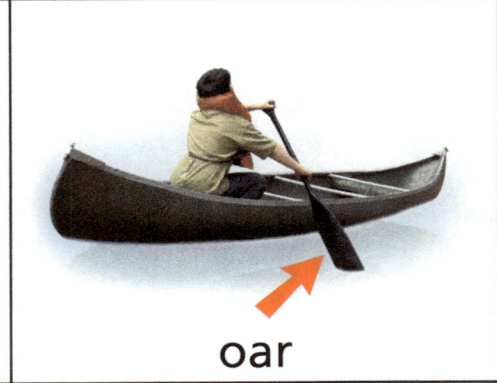 oar
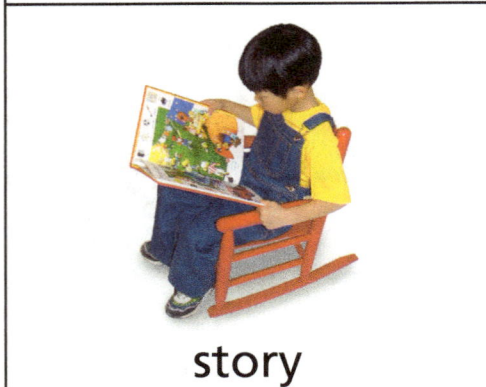 story	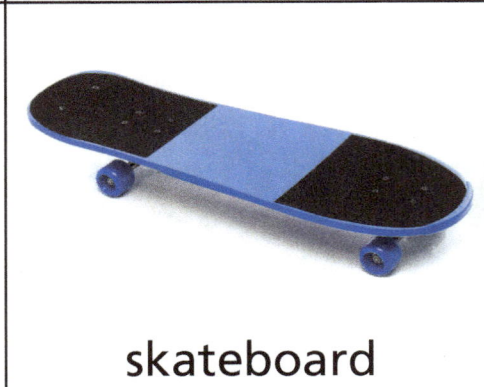 skateboard	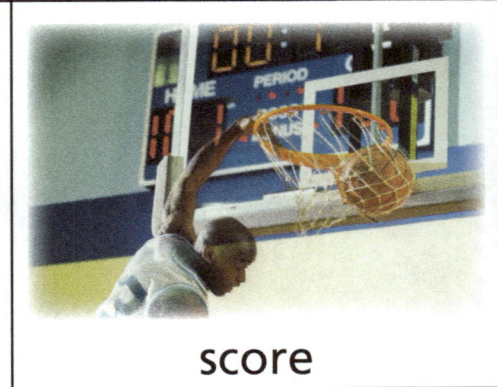 score

Name _____

Helper Signature _____

Speech - Language Pathologist _____

Date _____

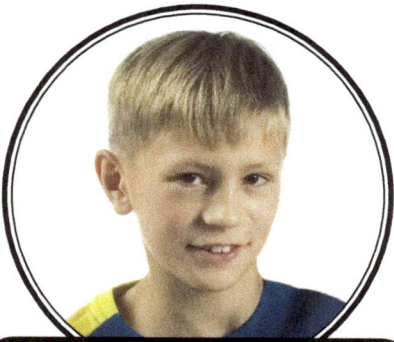

Barry

This is Barry. He carried all the things on this page.

R – Vocalic AIR

1. Practice your sound by saying the words on this page. (Ex. parachute, chariot, etc.). Say the last word twice.
2. Practice saying **Barry** with each of the words. (Ex. Barry parachute, Barry chariot, etc.). Say the last word pair twice.
3. Practice saying **carried** with these words. (Ex. Barry carried a parachute, etc.). Say one of the sentences twice.
4. Practice saying **spare** with these words. (Barry carried a spare parachute, etc.). Say one of the expanded sentences twice.

When you have finished this whole page you will have said your sound in 100 words! Good job!

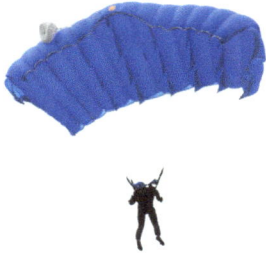 parachute	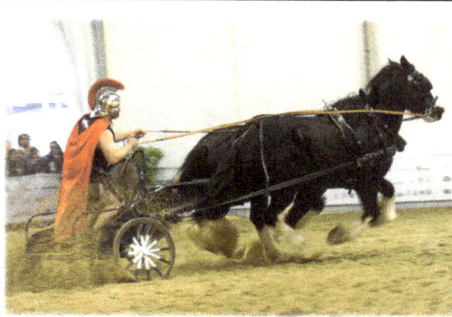 chariot	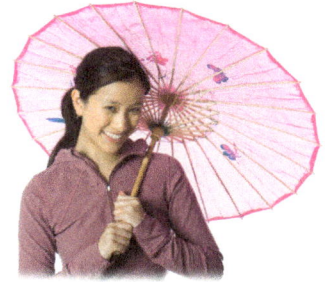 parasol
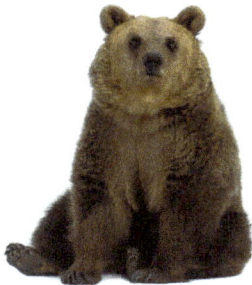 bear	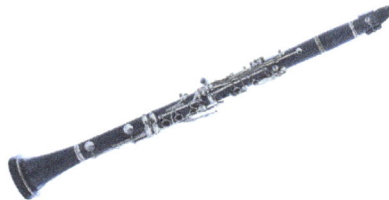 clarinet	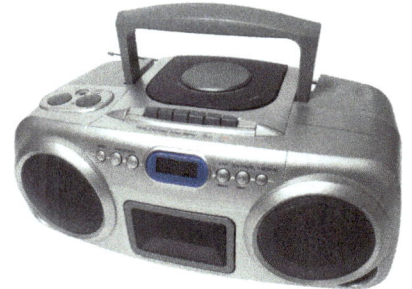 stereo
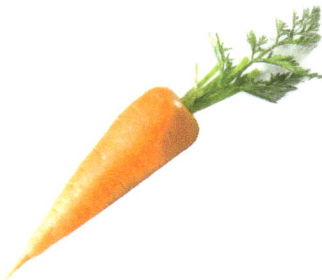 carrot	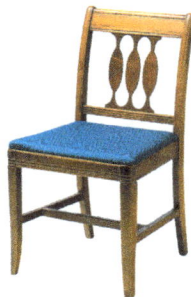 chair	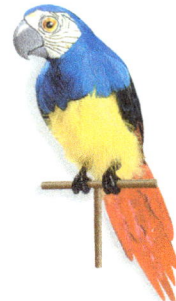 parrot

Name _____

Speech - Language Pathologist _____

Helper Signature _____

Date _____

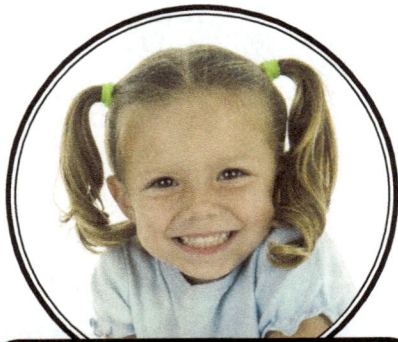

Claire

1. Practice your sound by saying the words on this page. (Ex. pear, parent, etc.). Say the last word twice.

2. Practice saying **Claire** with each of the words. (Ex. Claire pear, Claire parent, etc.). Say the last word pair twice.

3. Practice saying **cares about** with these words. (Ex. Claire cares about the pear, etc.). Say one of the sentences twice.

4. Practice saying **fair** with these words. (Claire cares about the fair pear, etc.). Say one of the expanded sentences twice.

This is Claire. She cares about all the things on this page.

When you have finished this whole page you will have said your sound in 100 words! Good job!

pear	parent	periscope
airplane	hair	mare
sparrow	square	cherries

Name

Helper Signature

Speech - Language Pathologist

Date

#BKCD-273 • *Say & Do® Artic Reps* • ©2015 Super Duper® Publications • www.superduperinc.com

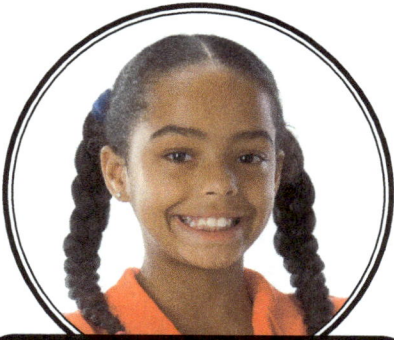

Keera

This is Keera. She can hear all the things on this page.

1. Practice your sound by saying the words on this page. (Ex. deer, cheer, etc.). Say the last word twice.

2. Practice saying **Keera** with each of the words. (Ex. Keera deer, Keera cheer, etc.). Say the last word pair twice.

3. Practice saying **can hear** with these words. (Ex. Keera can hear deer, etc.). Say one of the sentences twice.

4. Practice saying **nearby** with these words. (Keera can hear nearby deer, etc.). Say one of the expanded sentences twice.

When you have finished this whole page you will have said your sound in 100 words! Good job!

deer	cheer	gears
cashier	peers	spear
shears	cafeteria	hero

Name _____

Helper Signature _____

Speech - Language Pathologist _____

Date _____

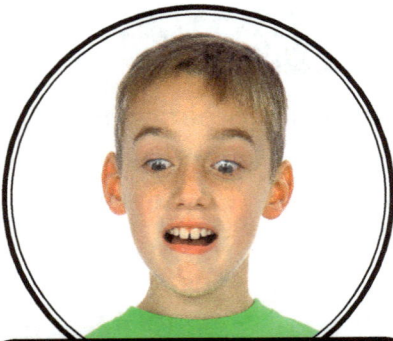

Pearce

This is Pearce. He fears all the things on this page.

R – Vocalic EAR

1. Practice your sound by saying the words on this page. (Ex. cereal, beard, etc.). Say the last word twice.

2. Practice saying **Pearce** with each of the words. (Ex. Pearce cereal, Pearce beard, etc.). Say the last word pair twice.

3. Practice saying **fears** with these words. (Ex. Pearce fears cereal, etc.). Say one of the sentences twice.

4. Practice saying **weird** with these words. (Pearce fears weird cereal, etc.). Say one of the expanded sentences twice.

When you have finished this whole page you will have said your sound in 100 words! Good job!

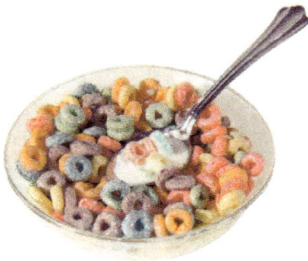 cereal	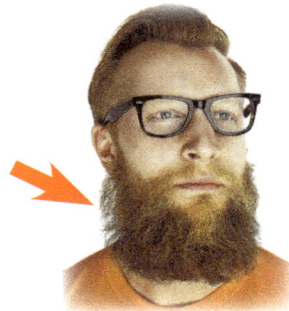 beard	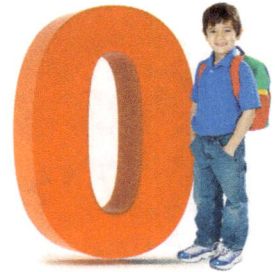 zero
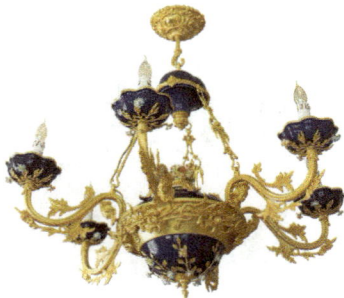 chandelier	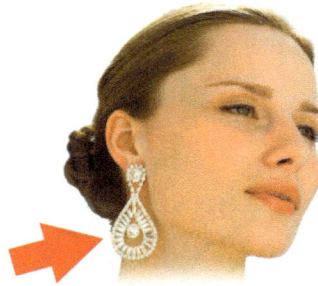 earring	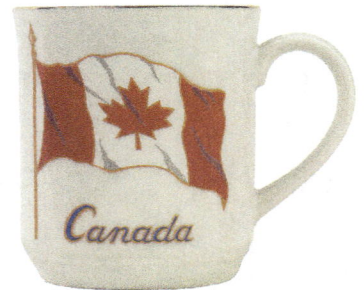 souvenir
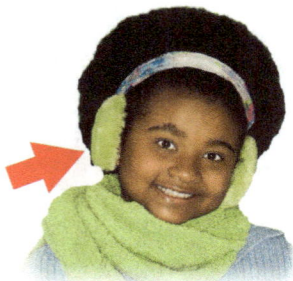 earmuffs	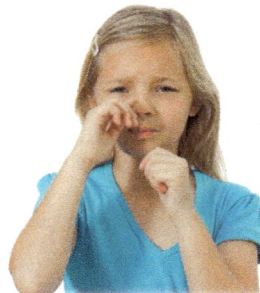 tears	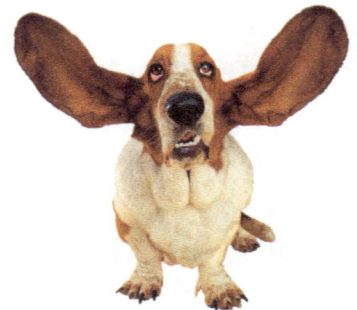 ears

Name _____

Helper Signature _____

Speech - Language Pathologist _____

Date _____

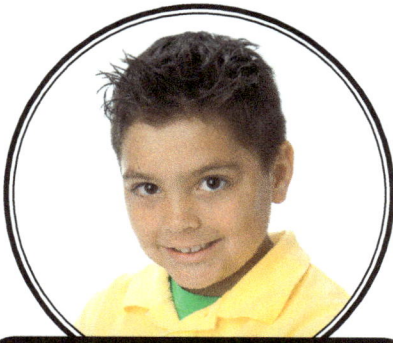

Maguire

This is Maguire. He admired all the things on this page.

R – Vocalic IRE

1. Practice your sound by saying the words on this page. (Ex. umpire, fire engine, etc.). Say the last word twice.

2. Practice saying **Maguire** with each of the words. (Ex. Maguire umpire, Maguire fire engine, etc.). Say the last word pair twice.

3. Practice saying **admired** with these words. (Ex. Maguire admired the umpire, etc.). Say one of the sentences twice.

4. Practice saying **tired** with these words. (Maguire admired the tired umpire, etc.). Say one of the expanded sentences twice.

When you have finished this whole page you will have said your sound in 100 words! Good job!

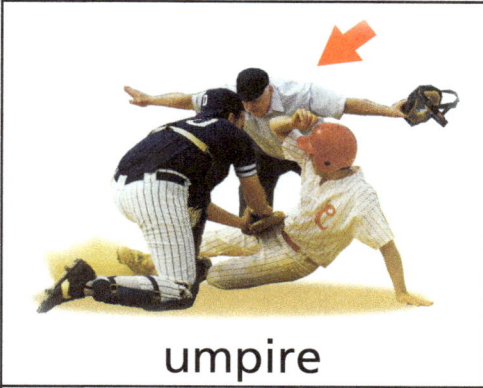 umpire	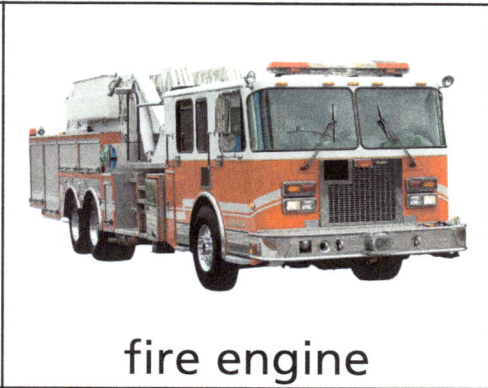 fire engine	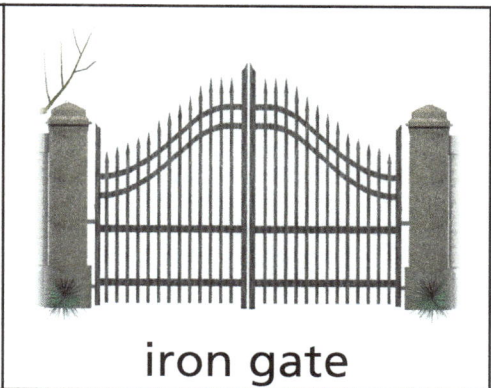 iron gate
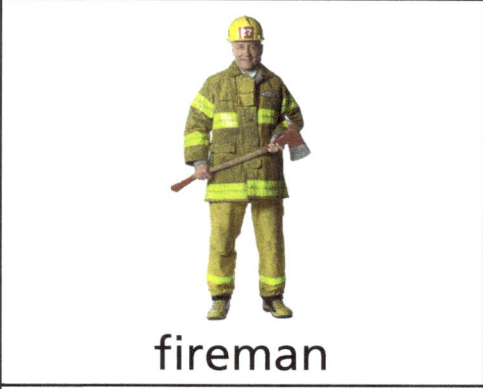 fireman	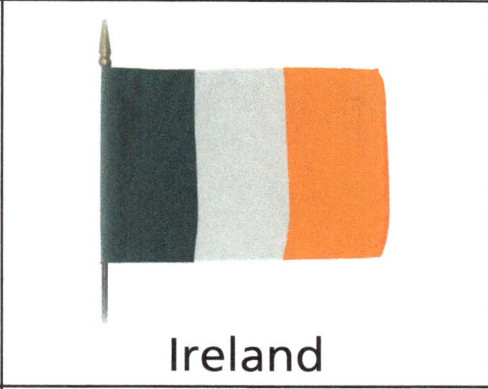 Ireland	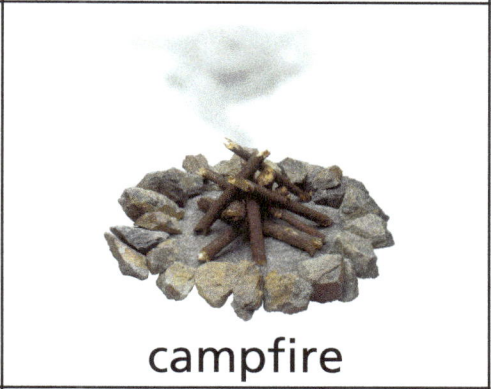 campfire
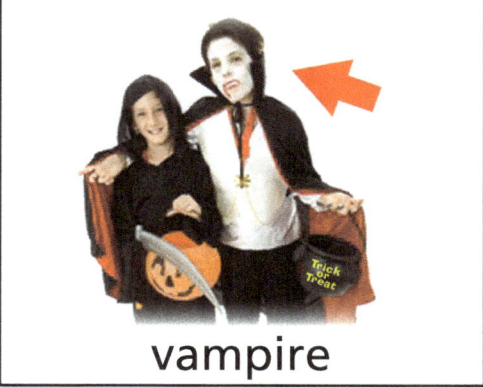 vampire	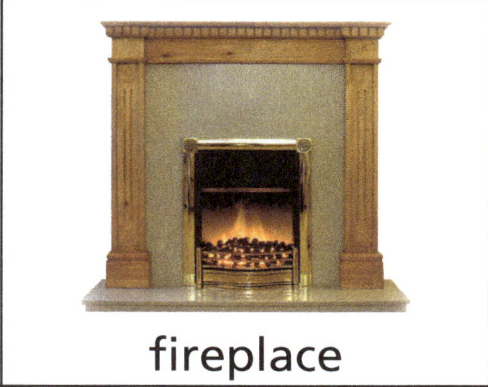 fireplace	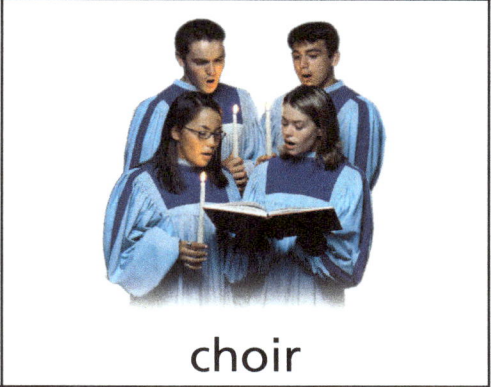 choir

Name _____

Helper Signature _____

Speech - Language Pathologist _____

Date _____

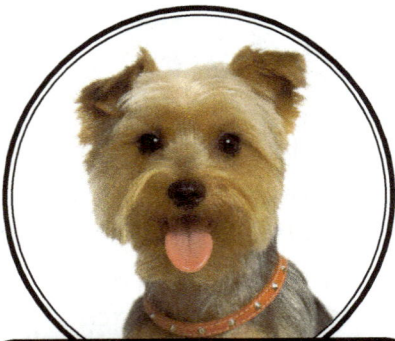

Fireball

This is Fireball. He acquires all the things on this page.

Vocalic IRE

1. Practice your sound by saying the words on this page. (Ex. sapphire, empire, etc.). Say the last word twice.

2. Practice saying **Fireball** with each of the words. (Ex. Fireball sapphire, Fireball empire, etc.). Say the last word pair twice.

3. Practice saying **acquires** with these words. (Ex. Fireball acquires the sapphire, etc.). Say one of the sentences twice.

4. Practice saying **entire** with these words. (Fireball acquires the entire sapphire, etc.). Say one of the **expanded** sentences twice.

When you have finished this whole page you will have said your sound in 100 words! Good job!

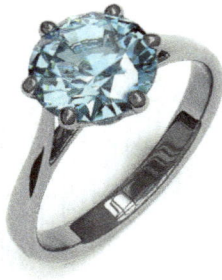 sapphire	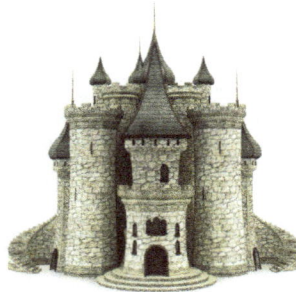 empire	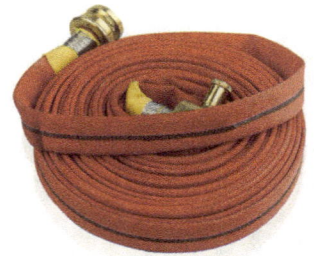 fire hose
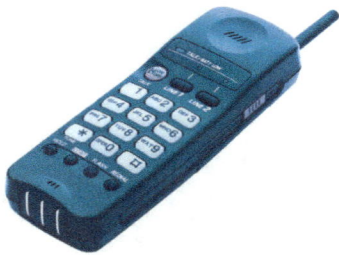 wireless phone	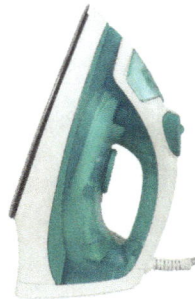 iron	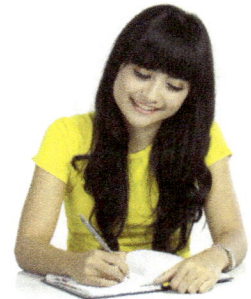 diary
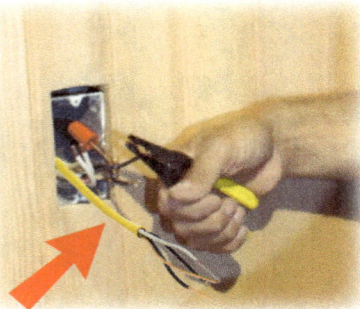 wire	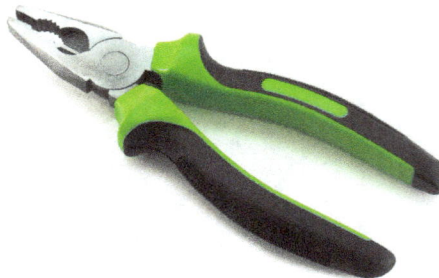 pliers	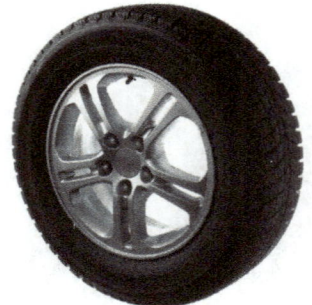 tire

Name _____

Helper Signature _____

Speech - Language Pathologist _____

Date _____

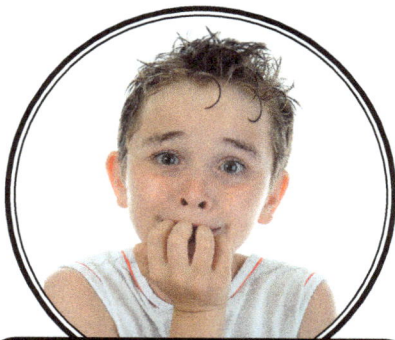

Brian

This is Brian. He broke all the things on this page.

BR – Blend

1. Practice your sound by saying the words on this page. (Ex. bread, brownies, etc.). Say the last word twice.
2. Practice saying **Brian** with each of the words. (Ex. Brian bread, Brian brownies, etc.). Say the last word pair twice.
3. Practice saying **broke** with these words. (Ex. Brian broke bread, etc.). Say one of the sentences twice.
4. Practice saying **brittle** with these words. (Brian broke brittle bread, etc.). Say one of the expanded sentences twice.

When you have finished this whole page you will have said your sound in 100 words! Good job!

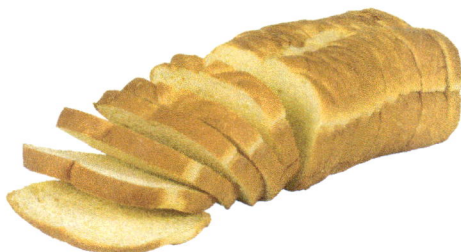 bread	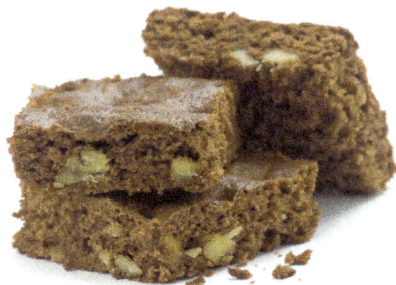 brownies	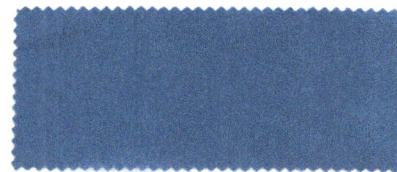 fabric
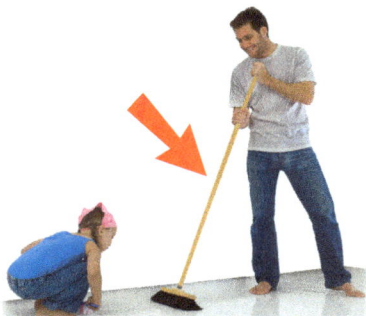 broom	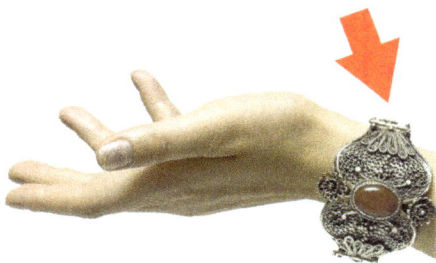 bracelet	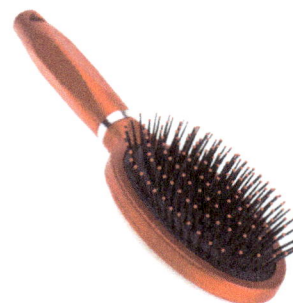 hairbrush
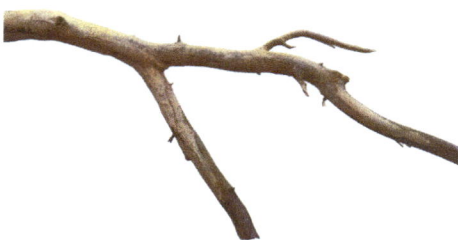 branch	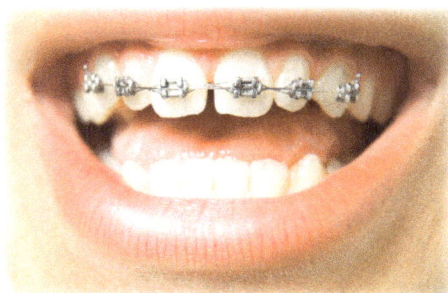 braces	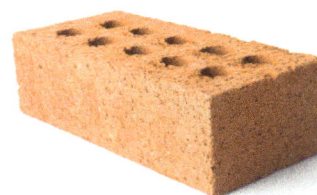 brick

Name _____

Speech - Language Pathologist _____

Helper Signature _____

Date _____

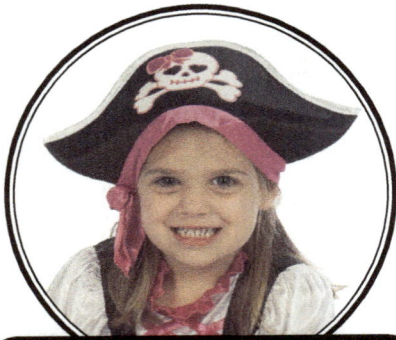

Brooke

This is Brooke. She brought all the things on this page.

BR – Blend

1. Practice your sound by saying the words on this page. (Ex. zebra, eyebrow, etc.). Say the last word twice.

2. Practice saying **Brooke** with each of the words. (Ex. Brooke zebra, Brooke eyebrow, etc.). Say the last word pair twice.

3. Practice saying **brought** with these words. (Ex. Brooke brought a zebra, etc.). Say one of the sentences twice.

4. Practice saying **brave** with these words. (Brooke brought the brave zebra, etc.). Say one of the expanded sentences twice.

When you have finished this whole page you will have said your sound in 100 words! Good job!

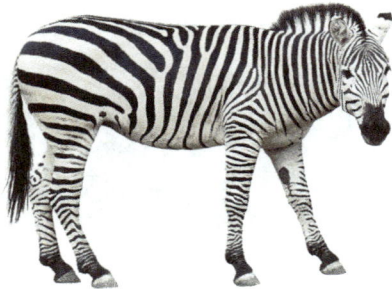 zebra	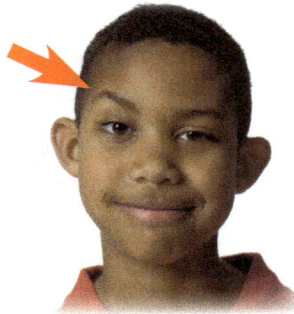 eyebrow	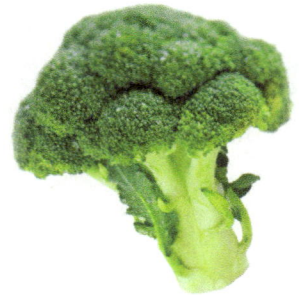 broccoli
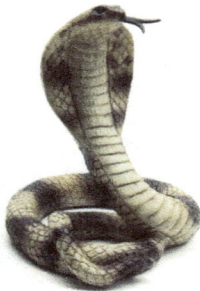 cobra	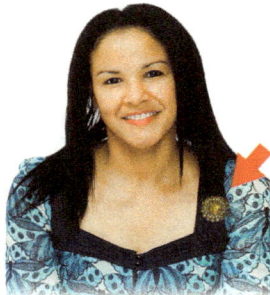 brooch	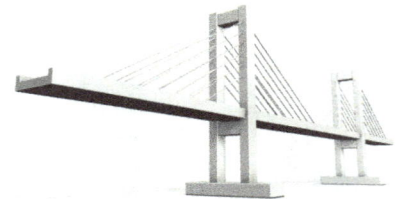 bridge
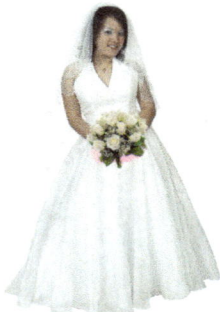 bride	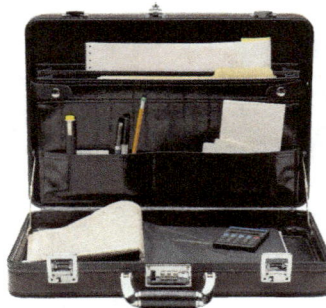 briefcase	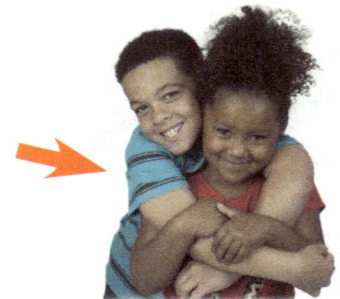 brother

Name _____

Helper Signature _____

Speech - Language Pathologist _____

Date _____

#BKCD-273 • *Say & Do® Artic Reps* • ©2015 Super Duper® Publications • www.superduperinc.com

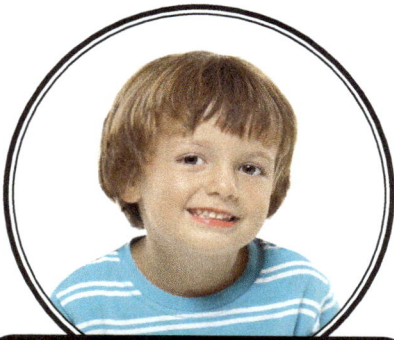

Drew

This is Drew. He dropped all the things on this page.

DR – Blend

1. Practice your sound by saying the words on this page. (Ex. drink, coughdrops, etc.). Say the last word twice.

2. Practice saying **Drew** with each of the words. (Ex. Drew drink, Drew coughdrops, etc.). Say the last word pair twice.

3. Practice saying **dropped** with these words. (Ex. Drew dropped the drink, etc.). Say one of the sentences twice.

4. Practice saying **dry** with these words. (Drew dropped a dry drink, etc.). Say one of the expanded sentences twice.

When you have finished this whole page you will have said your sound in 100 words! Good job!

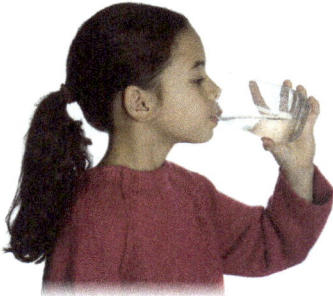

drink

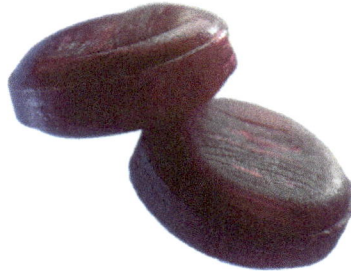

cough drops

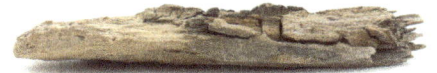

driftwood

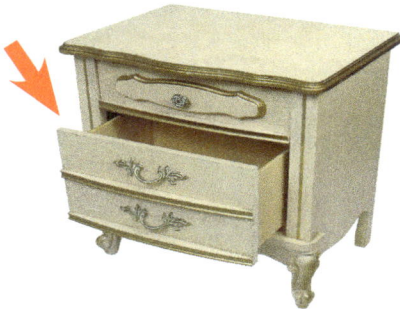

drawer

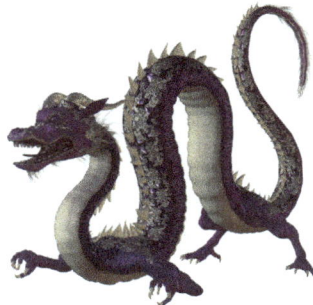

dragon

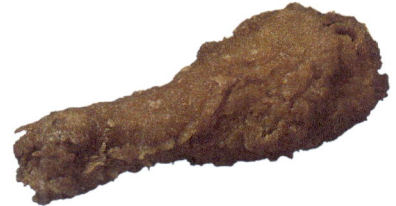

drumstick

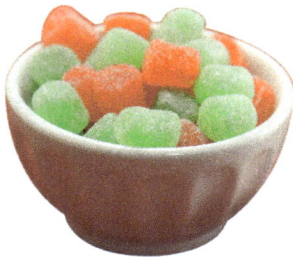

gumdrops

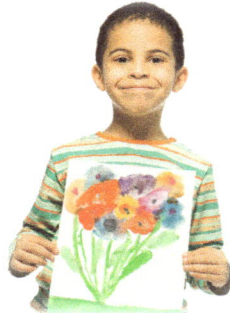

drawing

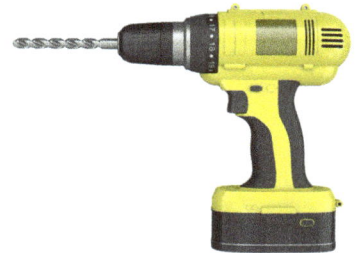

drill

Name

Helper Signature

Speech - Language Pathologist

Date

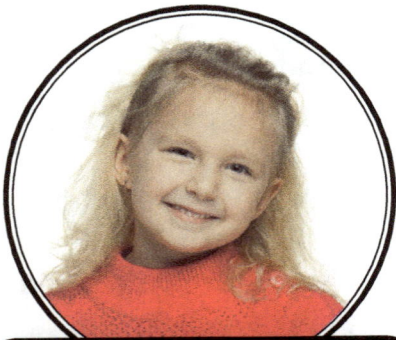

Audrey

This is Audrey. She dried all the things on this page.

DR – Blend

1. Practice your sound by saying the words on this page. (Ex. dress, driveway, etc.). Say the last word twice.

2. Practice saying **Audrey** with each of the words. (Ex. Audrey dress, Audrey driveway, etc.). Say the last word pair twice.

3. Practice saying **dried** with these words. (Ex. Audrey dried a dress, etc.). Say one of the sentences twice.

4. Practice saying **droopy** with these words. (Audrey dried a droopy dress, etc.). Say one of the expanded sentences twice.

   When you have finished this whole page you will have said your sound in 100 words! Good job!

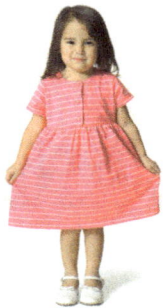 dress	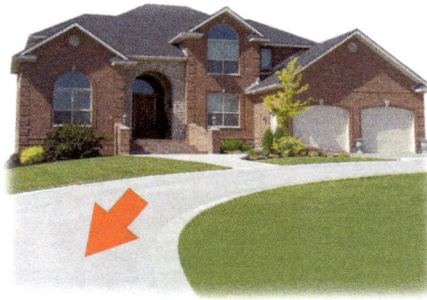 driveway	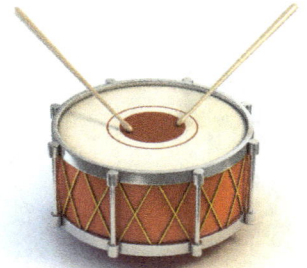 drum
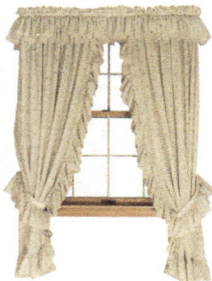 drapes	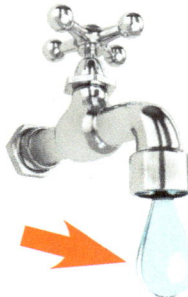 drop	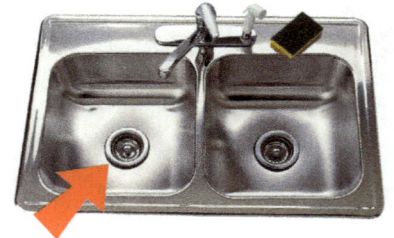 drain
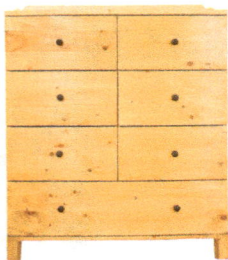 dresser	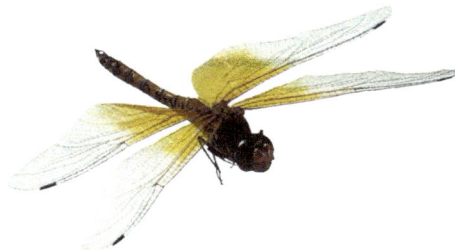 dragonfly	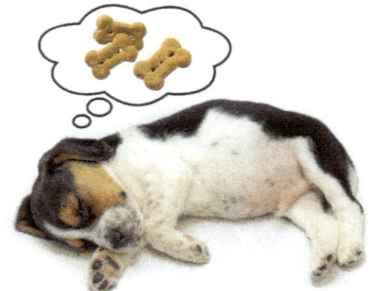 dream

Name _____

Helper Signature _____

Speech - Language Pathologist _____

Date _____

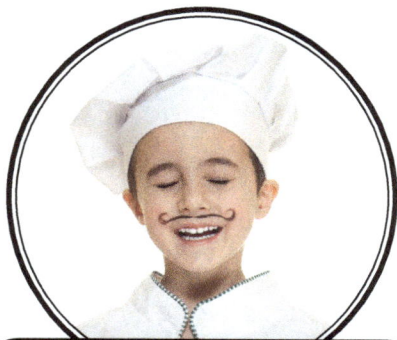

Fred

This is Fred. He fried all the things on this page.

FR – Blend

1. Practice your sound by saying the words on this page. (Ex. fruit, frisbee, etc.). Say the last word twice.
2. Practice saying **Fred** with each of the words. (Ex. Fred fruit, Fred frisbee, etc.). Say the last word pair twice.
3. Practice saying **fried** with these words. (Ex. Fred fried fruit, etc.). Say one of the sentences twice.
4. Practice saying **fresh** with these words. (Fred fried fresh fruit, etc.). Say one of the expanded sentences twice.

When you have finished this whole page you will have said your sound in 100 words! Good job!

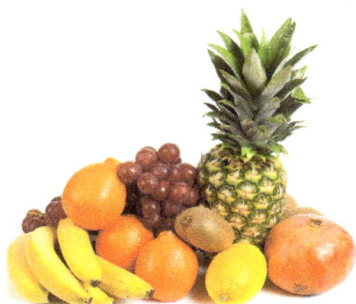

fruit

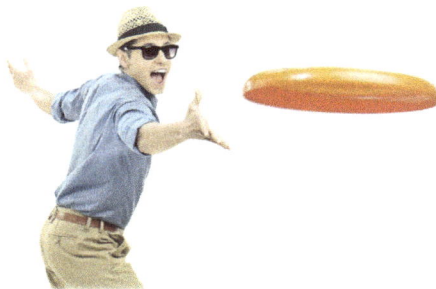

frisbee

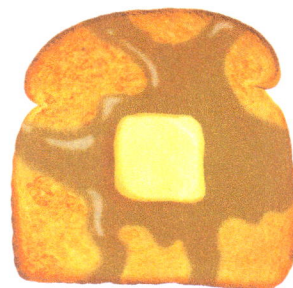

French toast

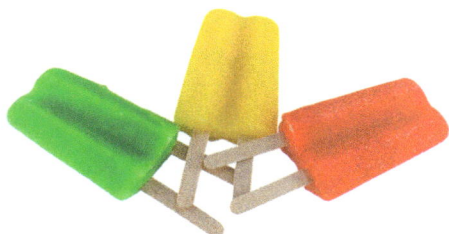

freezer pops

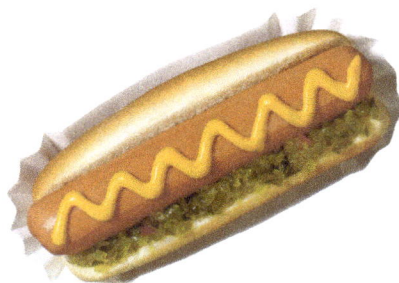

frankfurter

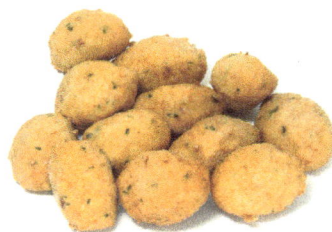

fritters

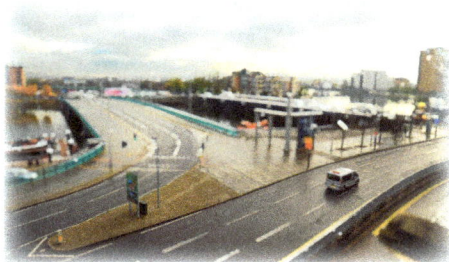

freeway

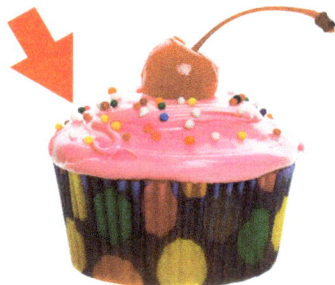

frosting

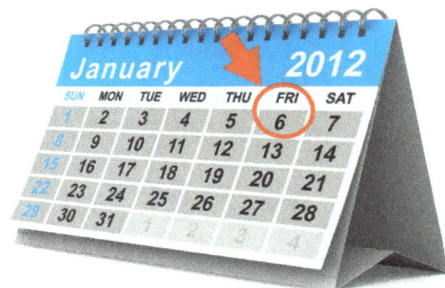

Friday

Name _____

Helper Signature _____

Speech - Language Pathologist _____

Date _____

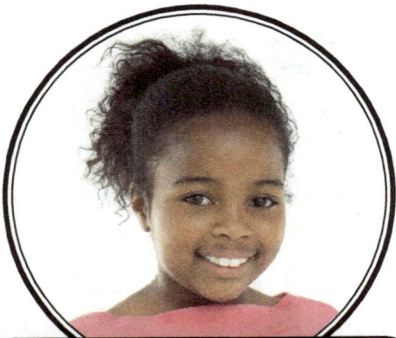

Frances

FR – Blend

This is Frances. She frightened all the things on this page.

1. Practice your sound by saying the words on this page. (Ex. friend, freezer, etc.). Say the last word twice.

2. Practice saying **Frances** with each of the words. (Ex. Frances friend, Frances freezer, etc.). Say the last word pair twice.

3. Practice saying **frightened** with these words. (Ex. Frances frightened a friend.). Say one of the sentences twice.

4. Practice saying **fragile** with these words. (Frances frightened a fragile friend, etc.). Say one of the expanded sentences twice.

When you have finished this whole page you will have said your sound in 100 words! Good job!

friend	freezer	fruit salad
freckles	frame	frog
frown	fraction	Frosty

Name _____

Speech - Language Pathologist _____

Helper Signature _____

Date _____

#BKCD-273 • *Say & Do® Artic Reps* • ©2015 Super Duper® Publications • www.superduperinc.com

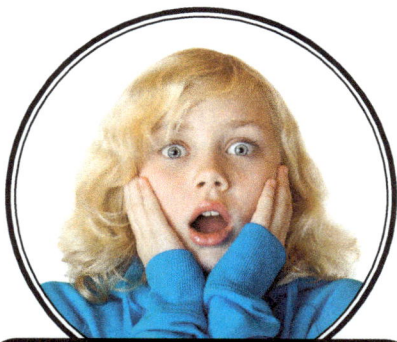

Gracie

This is Gracie. She grabbed all the things on this page.

GR – Blend

1. Practice your sound by saying the words on this page. (Ex. grapes, grill, etc.). Say the last word twice.

2. Practice saying **Gracie** with each of the words. (Ex. Gracie grapes, Gracie grill, etc.). Say the last word pair twice.

3. Practice saying **grabbed** with these words. (Ex. Gracie grabbed grapes, etc.). Say one of the sentences twice.

4. Practice saying **great** with these words. (Gracie grabbed great grapes, etc.). Say one of the expanded sentences twice.

When you have finished this whole page you will have said your sound in 100 words! Good job!

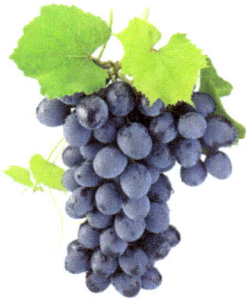 grapes	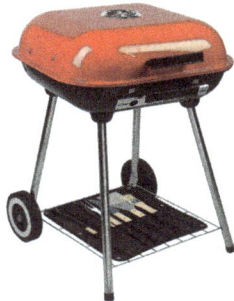 grill	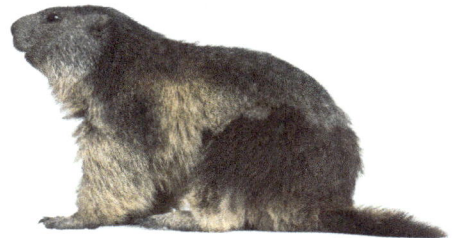 ground hog
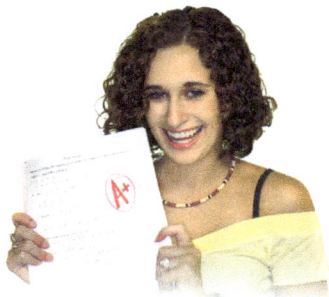 grade	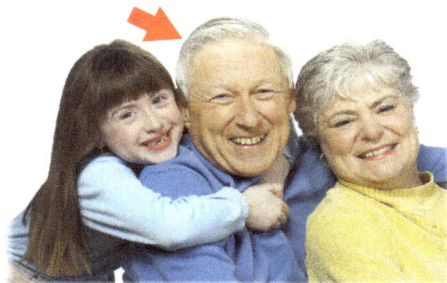 grandpa	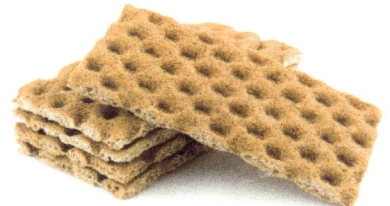 graham crackers
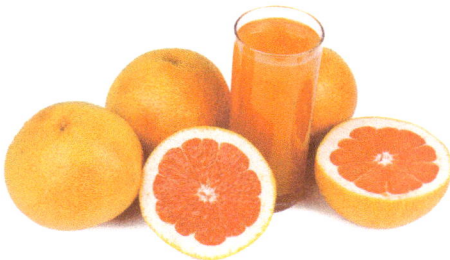 grapefruit	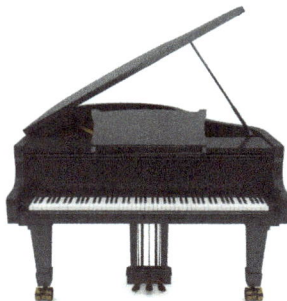 grand piano	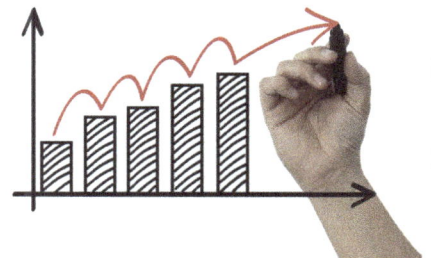 graph

Name _____

Speech - Language Pathologist _____

Helper Signature _____

Date _____

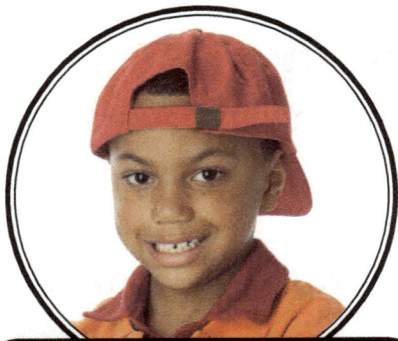

Grant

This is Grant. He greets all the things on this page.

GR – Blend

1. Practice your sound by saying the words on this page. (Ex. groom, grasshopper, etc.). Say the last word twice.

2. Practice saying **Grant** with each of the words. (Ex. Grant groom, Grant grasshopper, etc.). Say the last word pair twice.

3. Practice saying **greets** with these words. (Ex. Grant greets the groom.). Say one of the sentences twice.

4. Practice saying **grumpy** with these words. (Grant greets the grumpy groom, etc.). Say one of the expanded sentences twice.

When you have finished this whole page you will have said your sound in 100 words! Good job!

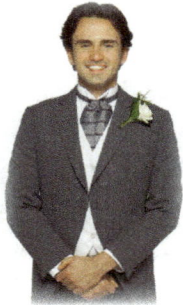 groom	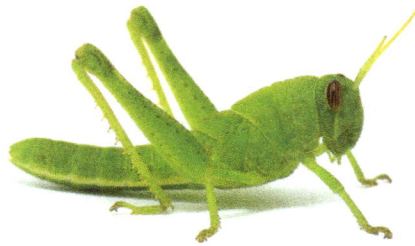 grasshopper	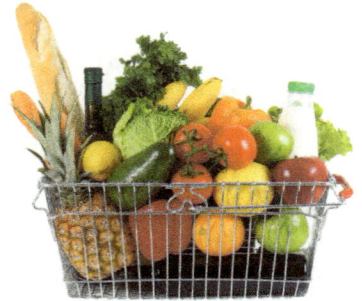 groceries
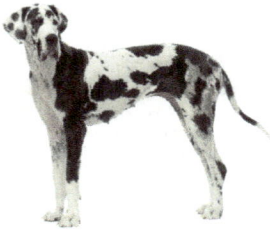 Great Dane	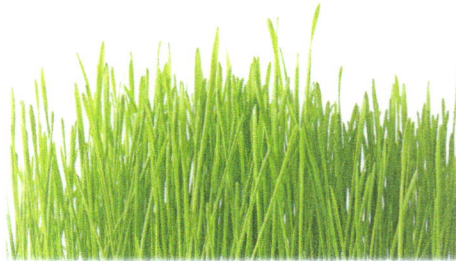 grass	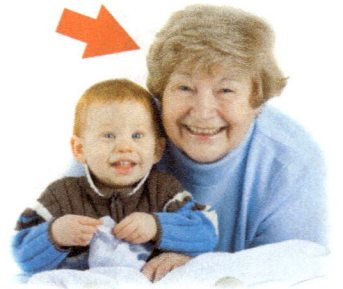 grandma
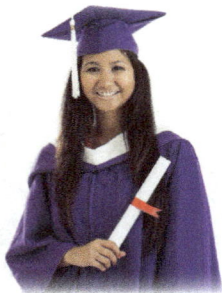 graduate	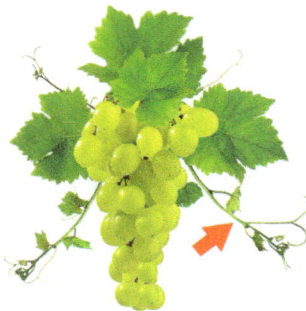 grapevine	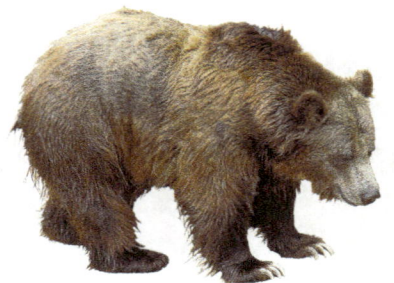 grizzly bear

Name _____

Speech - Language Pathologist _____

Helper Signature _____

Date _____

#BKCD-273 • *Say & Do® Artic Reps* • ©2015 Super Duper® Publications • www.superduperinc.com

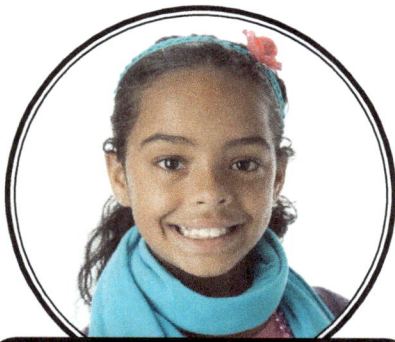

Kristin

This is Kristin. She crossed all the things on this page.

KR – Blend

1. Practice your sound by saying the words on this page. (Ex. creek, crab, etc.). Say the last word twice.

2. Practice saying **Kristin** with each of the words. (Ex. Kristin creek, Kristin crab, etc.). Say the last word pair twice.

3. Practice saying **crossed** with these words. (Ex. Kristin crossed the creek, etc.). Say one of the sentences twice.

4. Practice saying **crooked** with these words. (Kristin crossed a crooked creek, etc.). Say one of the expanded sentences twice.

When you have finished this whole page you will have said your sound in 100 words! Good job!

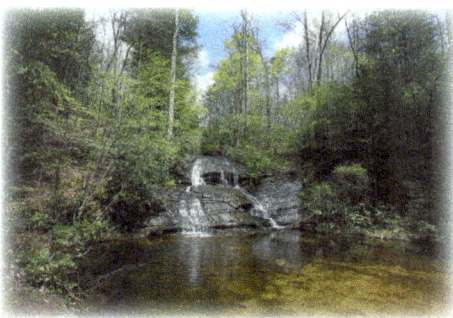 creek	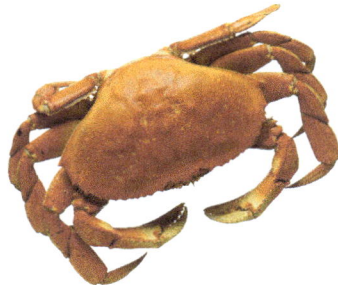 crab	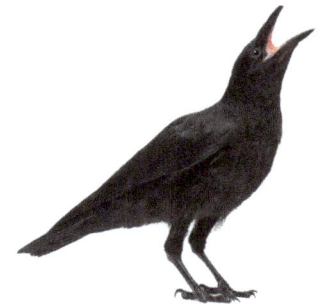 crow
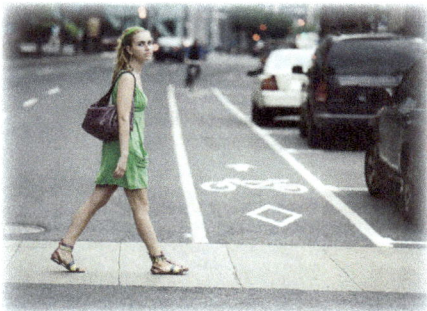 crosswalk	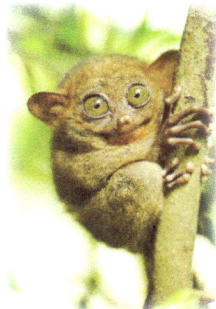 creature	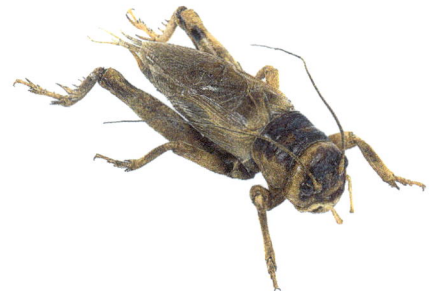 cricket
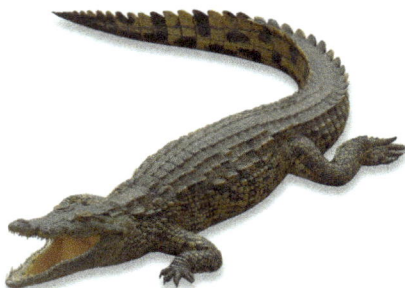 crocodile	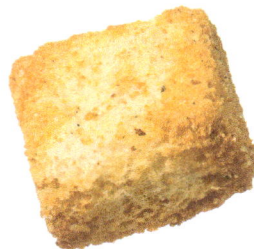 crouton	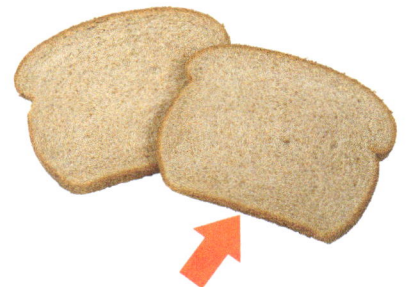 crust

Name _____

Helper Signature _____

Speech - Language Pathologist _____

Date _____

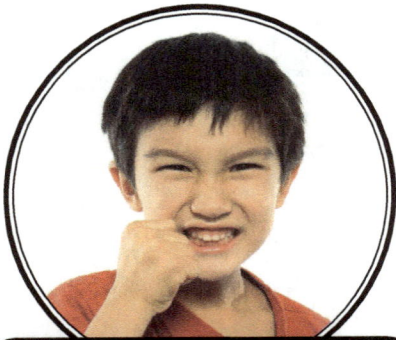

KR – Blend

1. Practice your sound by saying the words on this page. (Ex. crew, crown, etc.). Say the last word twice.

2. Practice saying **Chris** with each of the words. (Ex. Chris crew, Chris crown, etc.). Say the last word pair twice.

3. Practice saying **crushed** with these words. (Ex. Chris crushed the crew, etc.). Say one of the sentences twice.

4. Practice saying **crazy** with these words. (Chris crushed a crazy crew, etc.). Say one of the expanded sentences twice.

When you have finished this whole page you will have said your sound in 100 words! Good job!

Chris

This is Chris. He crushed all the things on this page.

crew	crown	crayons
cracker	cream	crib
crumbs	crane	cruise ship

Name _____

Helper Signature _____

Speech - Language Pathologist _____

Date _____

#BKCD-273 • *Say & Do*® Artic Reps • ©2015 Super Duper® Publications • www.superduperinc.com

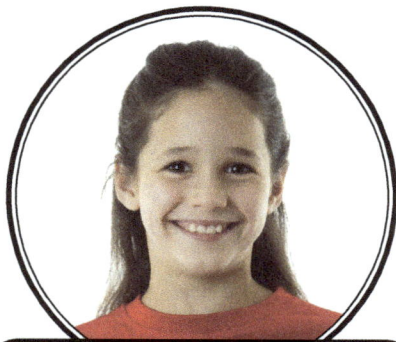

April

This is April. She pressed all the things on this page.

1. Practice your sound by saying the words on this page. (Ex. present, prince, etc.). Say the last word twice.

2. Practice saying **April** with each of the words. (Ex. April present, April prince, etc.). Say the last word pair twice.

3. Practice saying **pressed** with these words. (Ex. April pressed a present, etc.). Say one of the sentences twice.

4. Practice saying **priceless** with these words. (April pressed the priceless present, etc.). Say one of the expanded sentences twice.

When you have finished this whole page you will have said your sound in 100 words! Good job!

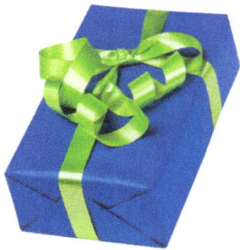 present	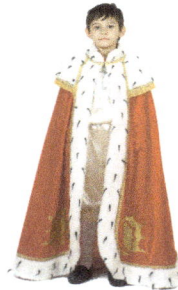 prince	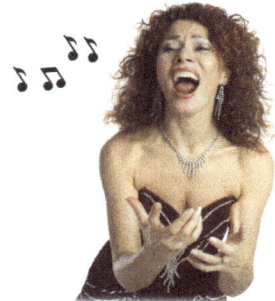 soprano
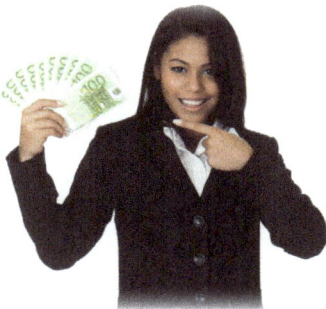 profit	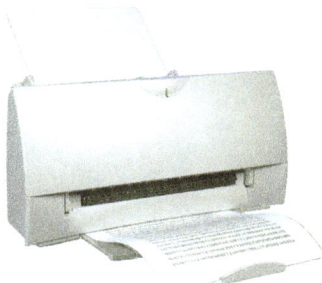 printer	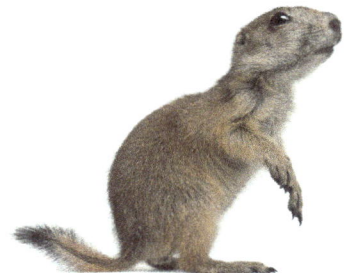 prairie dog
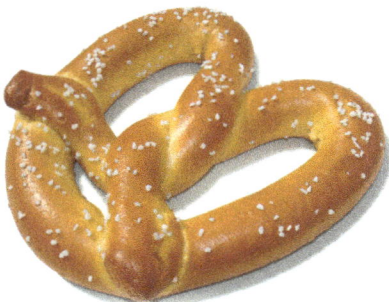 pretzel	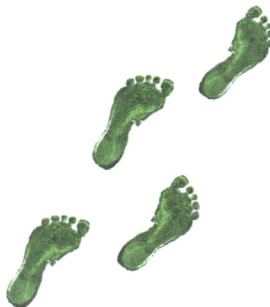 footprint	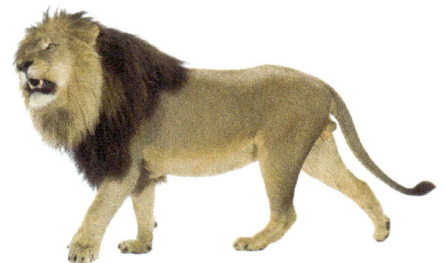 predator

Name _____

Helper Signature _____

Speech - Language Pathologist _____

Date _____

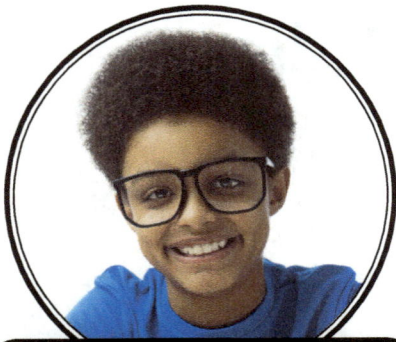

Preston

This is Preston. He prints all the things on this page.

1. Practice your sound by saying the words on this page. (Ex. prize, program, etc.). Say the last word twice.

2. Practice saying **Preston** with each of the words. (Ex. Preston prize, Preston program, etc.). Say the last word pair twice.

3. Practice saying **prints** with these words. (Ex. Preston prints the prize, etc.). Say one of the sentences twice.

4. Practice saying **prickly** with these words. (Preston prints a prickly prize, etc.). Say one of the expanded sentences twice.

When you have finished this whole page you will have said your sound in 100 words! Good job!

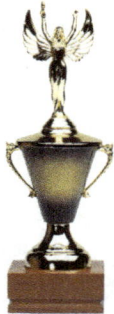 prize	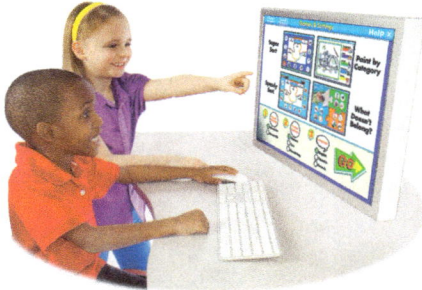 program	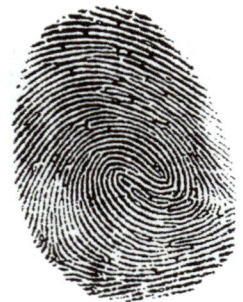 fingerprint
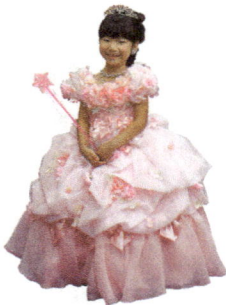 princess	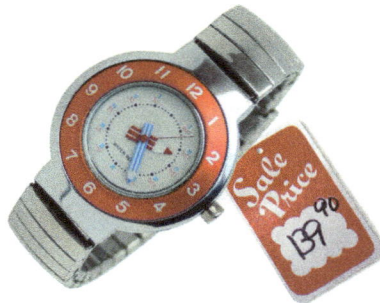 price	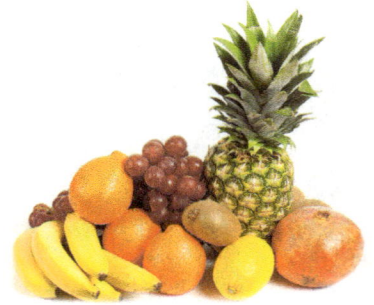 produce
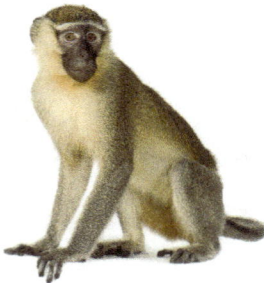 primate	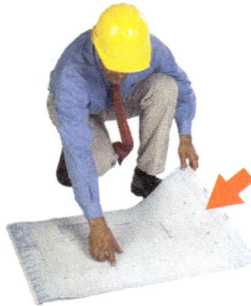 blueprint	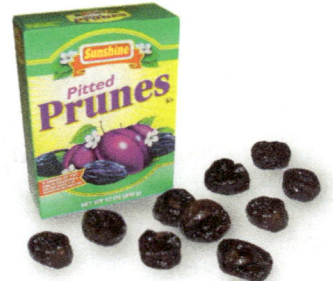 prune

Name _____

Speech - Language Pathologist _____

Helper Signature _____

Date _____

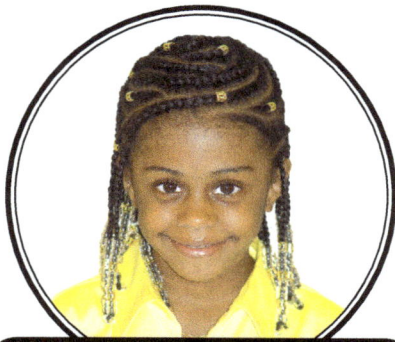

Tracy

This is Tracy. She tripped over all the things on this page.

1. Practice your sound by saying the words on this page. (Ex. track, treasure, etc.). Say the last word twice.

2. Practice saying **Tracy** with each of the words. (Ex. Tracy track, Tracy treasure, etc.). Say the last word pair twice.

3. Practice saying **tripped over** with these words. (Ex. Tracy tripped over the track, etc.). Say one of the sentences twice.

4. Practice saying **troublesome** with these words. (Tracy tripped over the troublesome track, etc.). Say one of the expanded sentences twice.

When you have finished this whole page you will have said your sound in 100 words! Good job!

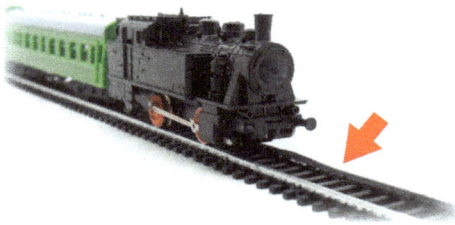

track

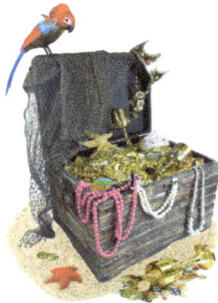

treasure

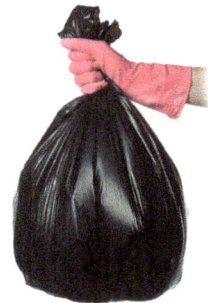

trash

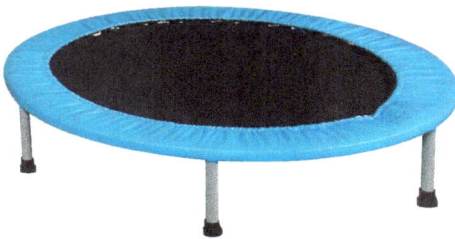

trampoline

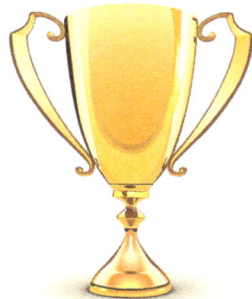

trophy

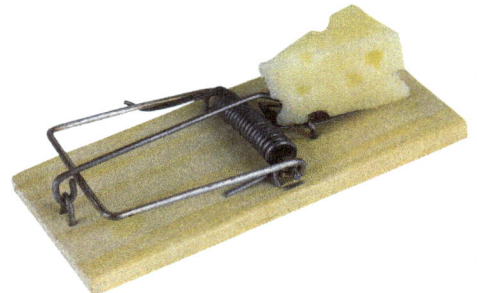

trap

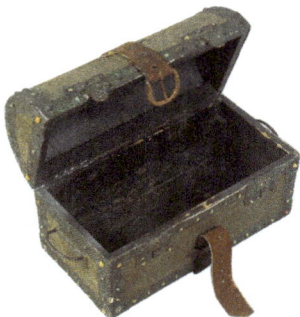

trunk

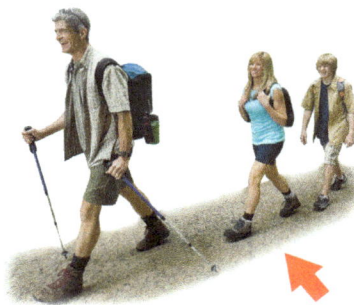

trail

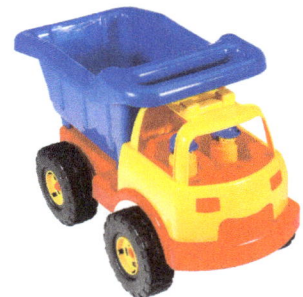

truck

Name _____

Helper Signature _____

Speech - Language Pathologist _____

Date _____

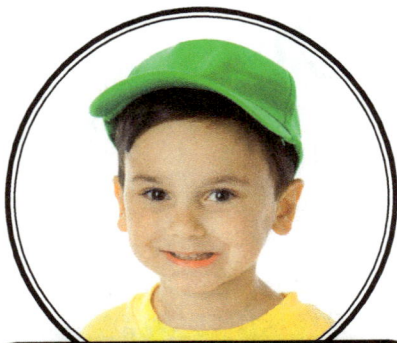

Trent

This is Trent. He traced all the things on this page.

TR – Blend

1. Practice your sound by saying the words on this page. (Ex. train, trick, etc.). Say the last word twice.

2. Practice saying **Trent** with each of the words. (Ex. Trent train, Trent trick, etc.). Say the last word pair twice.

3. Practice saying **traced** with these words. (Ex. Trent traced the train, etc.). Say one of the sentences twice.

4. Practice saying **tricky** with these words. (Trent traced the tricky train, etc.). Say one of the expanded sentences twice.

When you have finished this whole page you will have said your sound in 100 words! Good job!

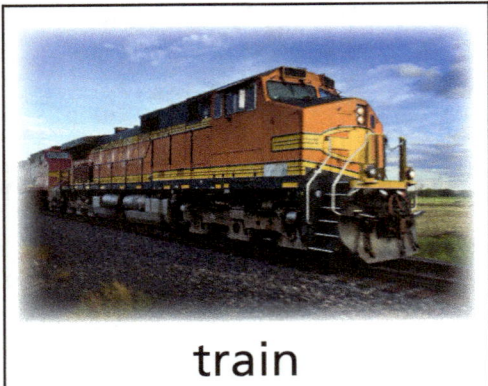 train	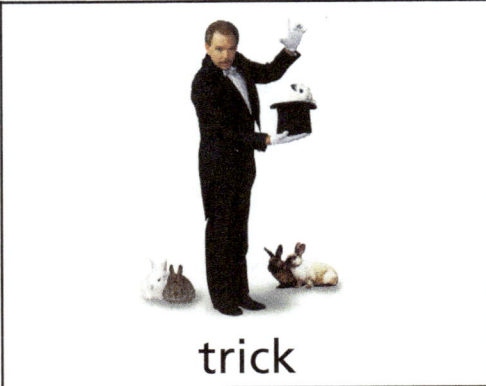 trick	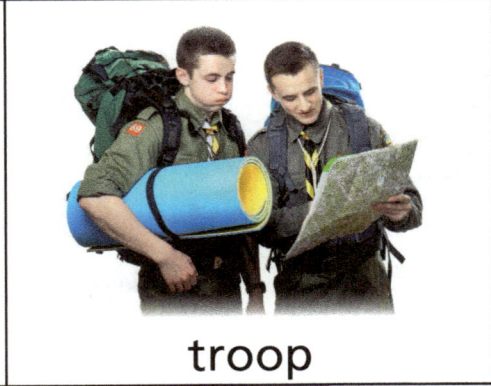 troop
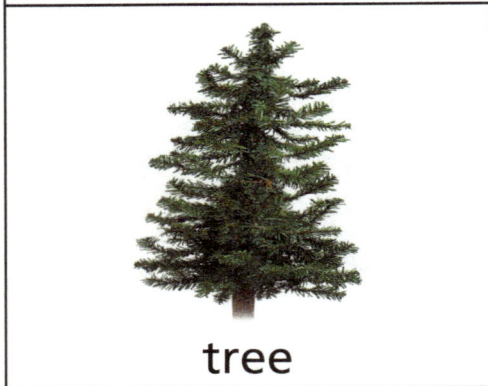 tree	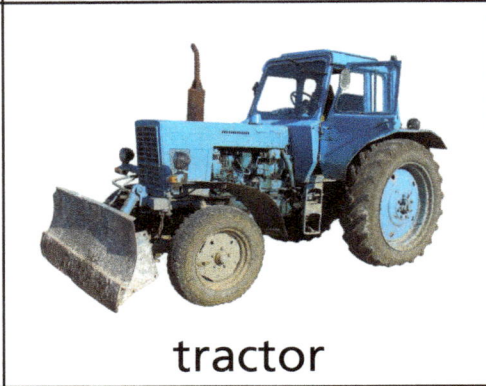 tractor	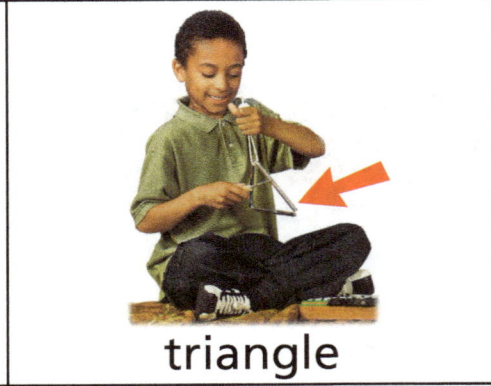 triangle
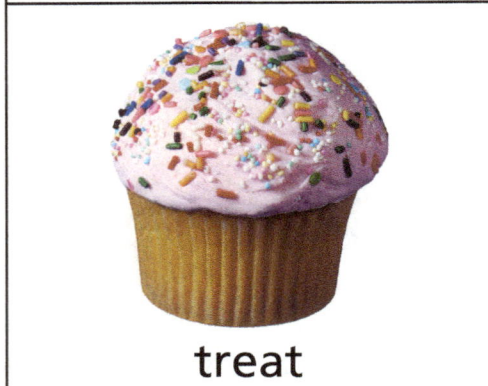 treat	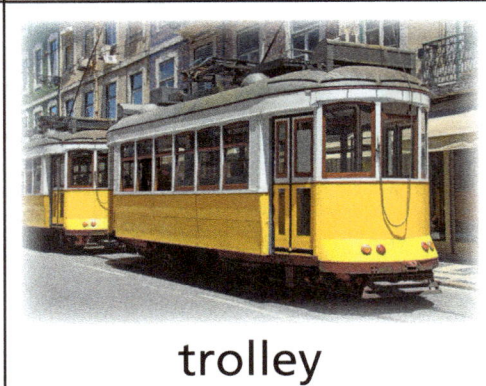 trolley	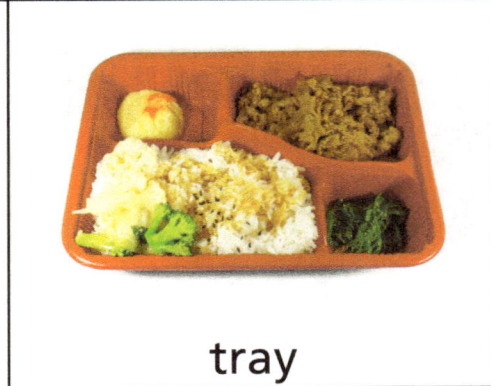 tray

Name _____

Helper Signature _____

Speech - Language Pathologist _____

Date _____

#BKCD-273 • *Say & Do® Artic Reps* • ©2015 Super Duper® Publications • www.superduperinc.com

S

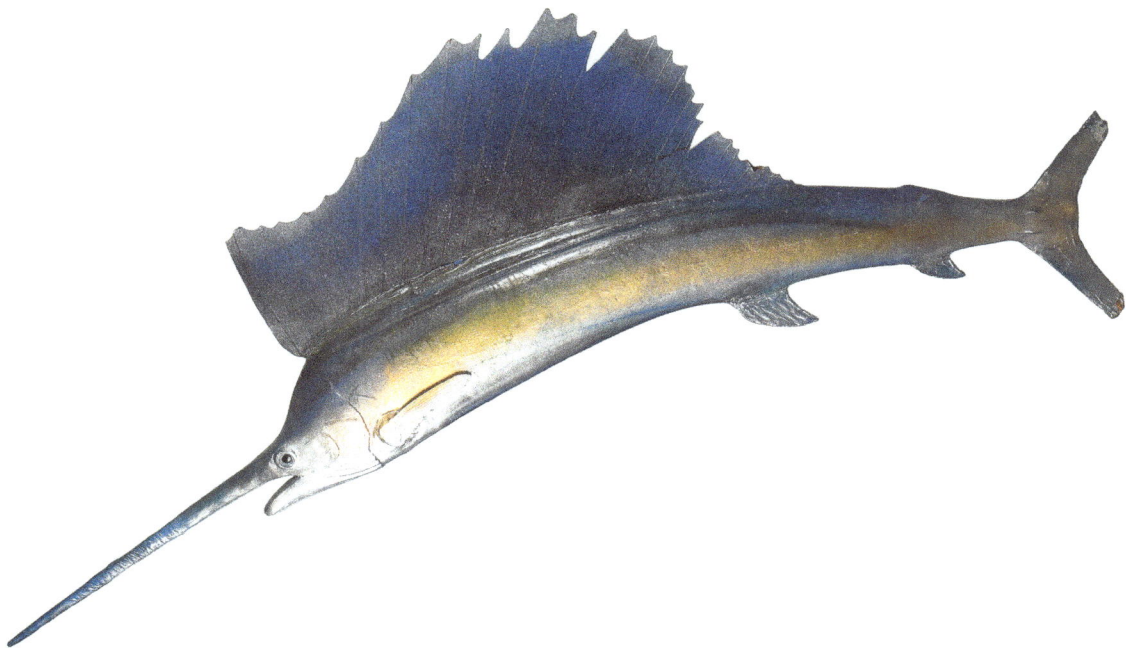

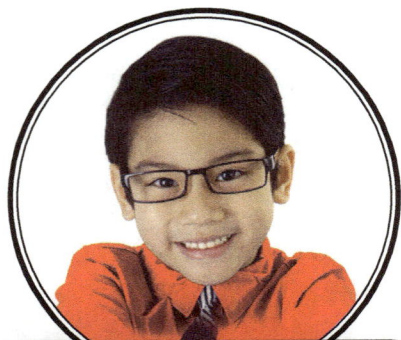

Sam

This is Sam. He saw all the things on this page.

S – Initial Position

1. Practice your sound by saying the words on this page. (Ex. Santa, sailboat, etc.). Say the last word twice.

2. Practice saying **Sam** with each of the words. (Ex. Sam Santa, Sam sailboat, etc.). Say the last word pair twice.

3. Practice saying **saw** with these words. (Ex. Sam saw Santa, etc.). Say one of the sentences twice.

4. Practice saying **satin** with these words. (Sam saw a satin Santa, etc.). Say one of the expanded sentences twice.

When you have finished this whole page you will have said your sound in 100 words! Good job!

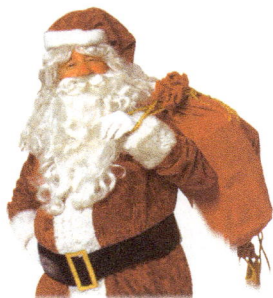 Santa	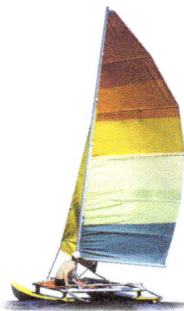 sailboat	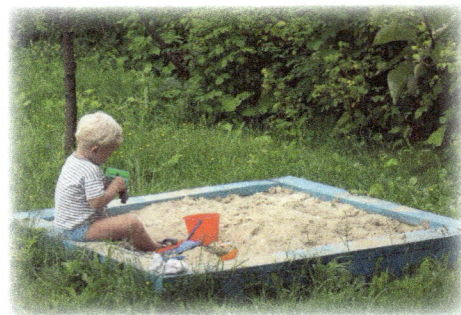 sandbox
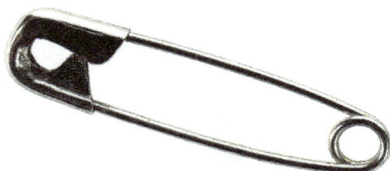 safety pin	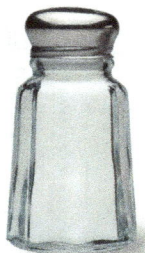 salt	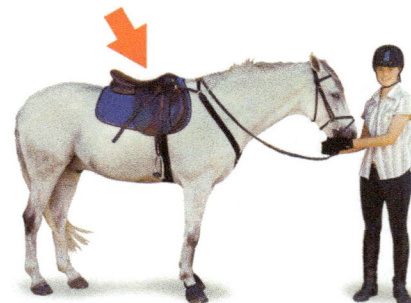 saddle
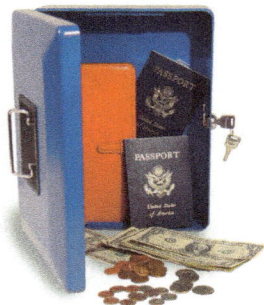 safe	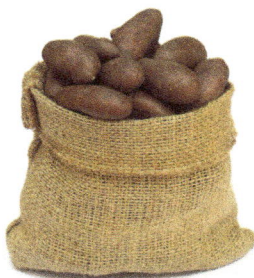 sack	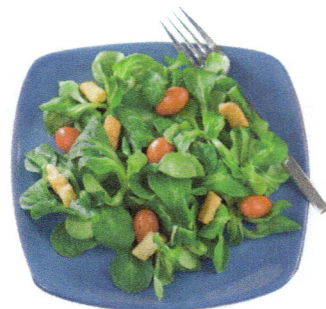 salad

Name _____

Speech - Language Pathologist _____

Helper Signature _____

Date _____

#BKCD-273 • *Say & Do® Artic Reps* • ©2015 Super Duper® Publications • www.superduperinc.com

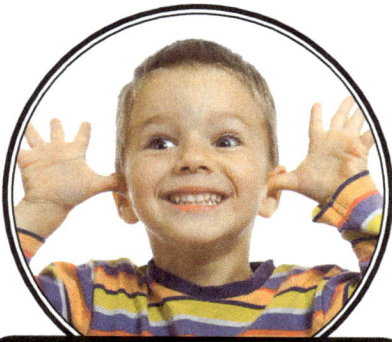

Cedric

This is Cedric. He sent all the things on this page.

S – Initial Position

1. Practice your sound by saying the words on this page. (Ex. sea, seat, etc.). Say the last word twice.
2. Practice saying **Cedric** with each of the words. (Ex. Cedric sea, Cedric seat, etc.). Say the last word pair twice.
3. Practice saying **sent** with these words. (Ex. Cedric sent a sea, etc.). Say one of the sentences twice.
4. Practice saying **sandy** with these words. (Cedric sent a sandy sea, etc.). Say one of the expanded sentences twice.

When you have finished this whole page you will have said your sound in 100 words! Good job!

sea	seat	seatbelt
sea lion	cereal	sewing machine
celebrity	celery	ceiling

Name _____

Helper Signature _____

Speech - Language Pathologist _____

Date _____

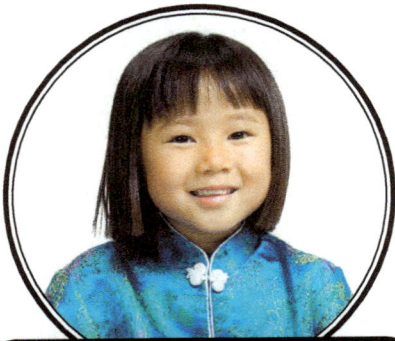

Cindy

This is Cindy. She will sit on all the things on this page.

1. Practice your sound by saying the words on this page. (Ex. sign, circle, etc.). Say the last word twice.

2. Practice saying **Cindy** with each of the words. (Ex. Cindy sign, Cindy circle, etc.). Say the last word pair twice.

3. Practice saying **will sit on** with these words. (Ex. Cindy will sit on a sign, etc.). Say one of the sentences twice.

4. Practice saying **silver** with these words. (Cindy will sit on a silver sign, etc.). Say one of the expanded sentences twice.

When you have finished this whole page you will have said your sound in 100 words! Good job!

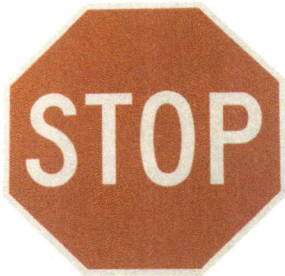 sign	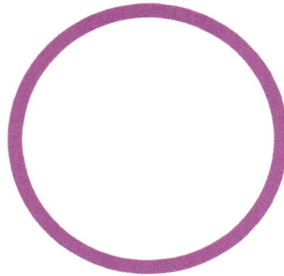 circle	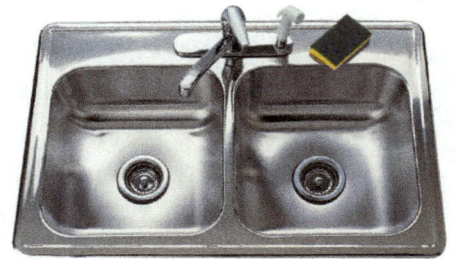 sink
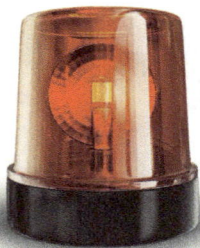 siren	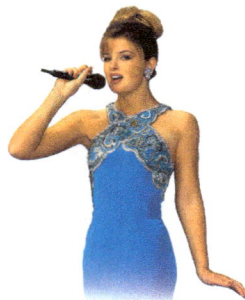 singer	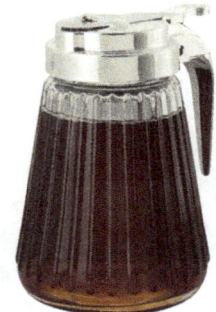 syrup
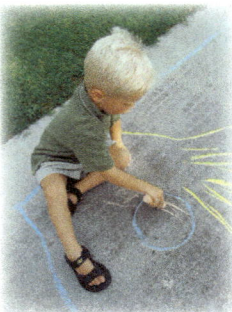 sidewalk	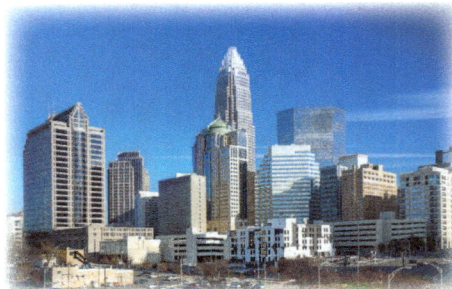 city	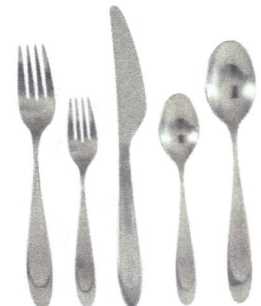 silverware

Name _____

Helper Signature _____

Speech - Language Pathologist _____

Date _____

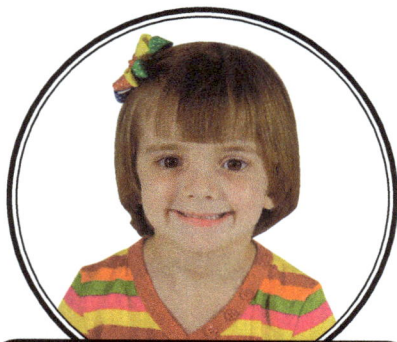

Sophie

This is Sophie. She sold all the things on this page.

1. Practice your sound by saying the words on this page. (Ex. soap, sock, etc.). Say the last word twice.

2. Practice saying **Sophie** with each of the words. (Ex. Sophie soap, Sophie sock, etc.). Say the last word pair twice.

3. Practice saying **sold** with these words. (Ex. Sophie sold soap, etc.). Say one of the sentences twice.

4. Practice saying **soft** with these words. (Sophie sold soft soap, etc.). Say one of the expanded sentences twice.

When you have finished this whole page you will have said your sound in 100 words! Good job!

soap	sock	soda
soup	soccer ball	sofa
soil	swordfish	sword

Name _____

Helper Signature _____

Speech - Language Pathologist _____

Date _____

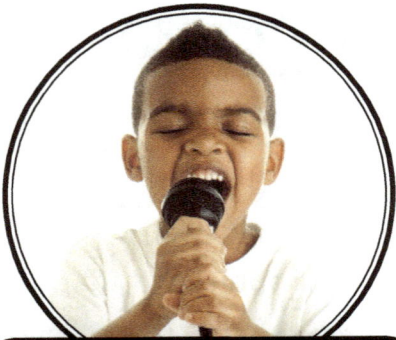

Sonny

This is Sonny. He sang about all the things on this page.

S – Initial Position

1. Practice your sound by saying the words on this page. (Ex. supermarket, sun, etc.). Say the last word twice.

2. Practice saying **Sonny** with each of the words. (Ex. Sonny supermarket, Sonny sun, etc.). Say the last word pair twice.

3. Practice saying **sang about** with these words. (Ex. Sonny sang about the supermarket, etc.). Say one of the sentences twice.

4. Practice saying **super** with these words. (Sonny sang about the super supermarket, etc.). Say one of the expanded sentences twice.

When you have finished this whole page you will have said your sound in 100 words! Good job!

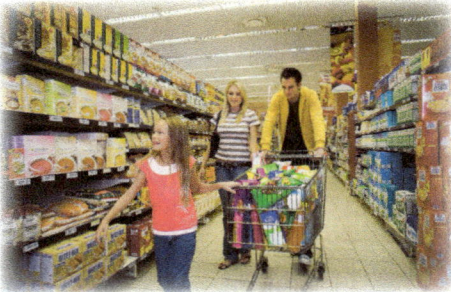 supermarket	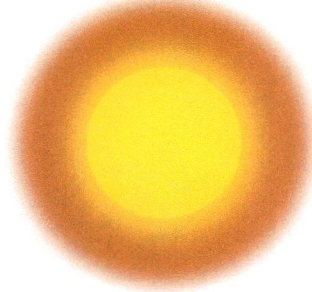 sun	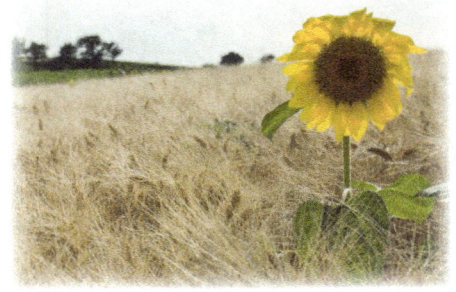 sunflower
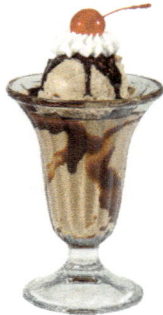 sundae	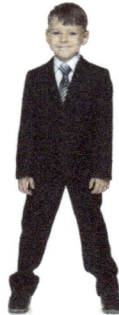 suit	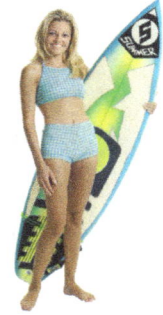 surfboard
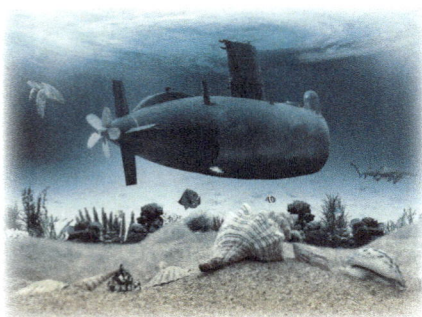 submarine	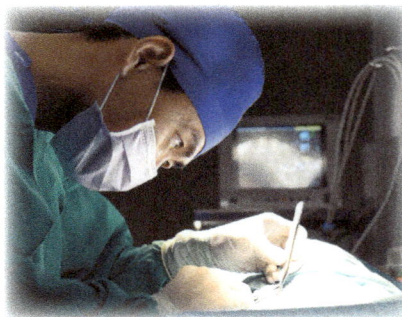 surgeon	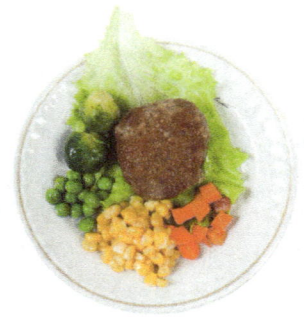 supper

Name _____

Helper Signature _____

Speech - Language Pathologist _____

Date _____

#BKCD-273 • *Say & Do® Artic Reps* • ©2015 Super Duper® Publications • www.superduperinc.com

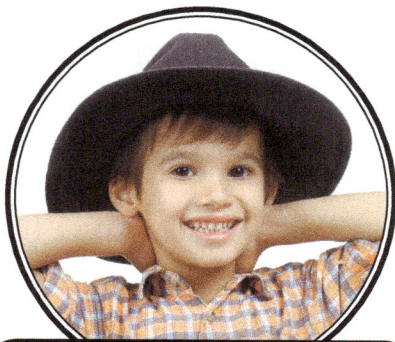

Jason

This is Jason. He was facing all the things on this page.

S – Medial Position

1. Practice your sound by saying the words on this page. (Ex. recipe, blossom, etc.). Say the last word twice.

2. Practice saying **Jason** with each of the words. (Ex. Jason recipe, Jason blossom, etc.). Say the last word pair twice.

3. Practice saying **was facing** with these words. (Ex. Jason was facing the recipe, etc.). Say one of the sentences twice.

4. Practice saying **juicy** with these words. (Jason was facing a juicy recipe, etc.). Say one of the expanded sentences twice.

When you have finished this whole page you will have said your sound in 100 words! Good job!

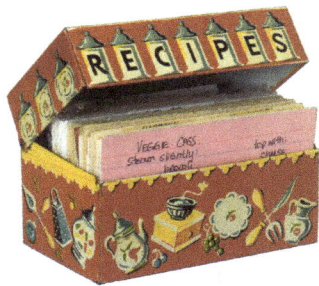 recipe	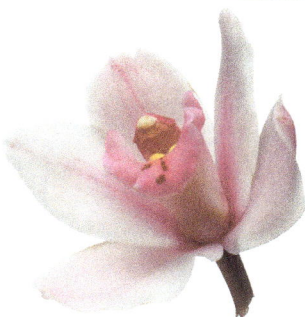 blossom	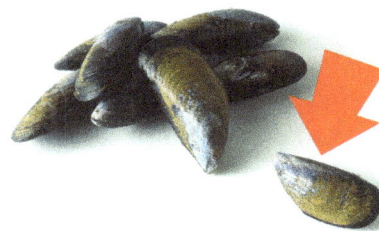 mussel
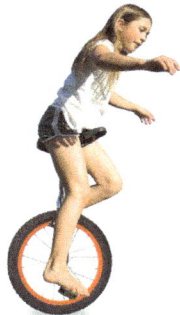 unicycle	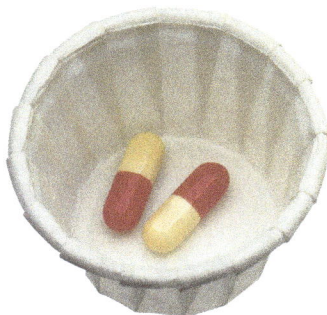 medicine	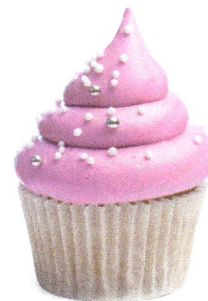 icing
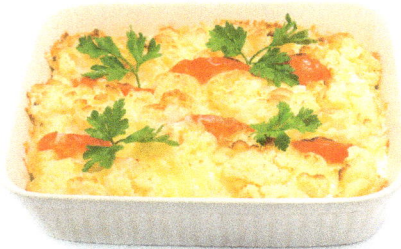 casserole	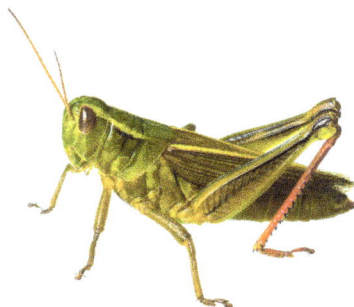 grasshopper	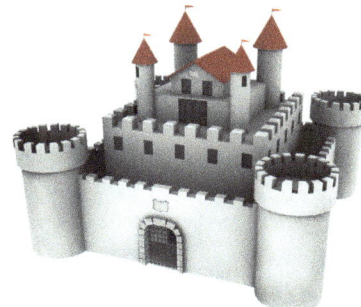 castle

Name _____

Helper Signature _____

Speech - Language Pathologist _____

Date _____

S – Medial Position

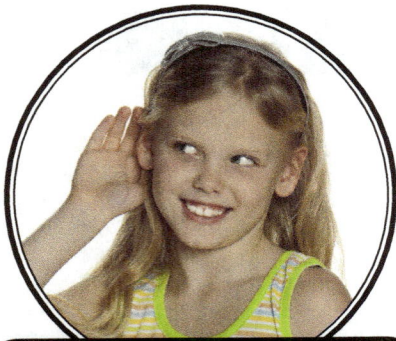

Missy

This is Missy. She listened to all the things on this page.

1. Practice your sound by saying the words on this page. (Ex. motorcycle, hairdresser, etc.). Say the last word twice.

2. Practice saying **Missy** with each of the words. (Ex. Missy motorcycle, Missy hairdresser, etc.). Say the last word pair twice

3. Practice saying **listened to** with these words. (Ex. Missy listened to the motorcycle, etc.). Say one of the sentences twice.

4. Practice saying **bossy** with these words. (Missy listened to the bossy motorcycle, etc.). Say one of the expanded sentences twice

When you have finished this whole page you will have said your sound in 100 words! Good job!

motorcycle	hairdresser	lasso
insect	faucet	receipt
passengers	principal	dinosaur

Name _____

Helper Signature _____

Speech - Language Pathologist _____

Date _____

#BKCD-273 • *Say & Do® Artic Reps* • ©2015 Super Duper® Publications • www.superduperinc.com

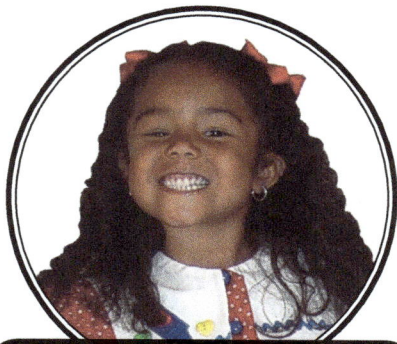

Lucy

This is Lucy. She was loosening all the things on this page.

S – Medial Position

1. Practice your sound by saying the words on this page. (Ex. glasses, gasoline, etc.). Say the last word twice.

2. Practice saying **Lucy** with each of the words. (Ex. Lucy glasses, Lucy gasoline, etc.). Say the last word pair twice.

3. Practice saying **was loosening** with these words. (Ex. Lucy was loosening the glasses, etc.). Say one of the sentences twice.

4. Practice saying **awesome** with these words. (Lucy was loosening the awesome glasses, etc.). Say one of the expanded sentences twice.

When you have finished this whole page you will have said your sound in 100 words! Good job!

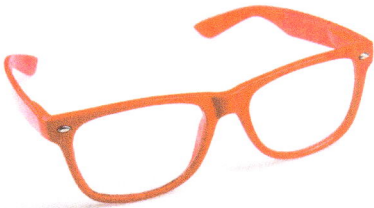 glasses	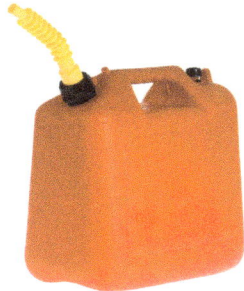 gasoline	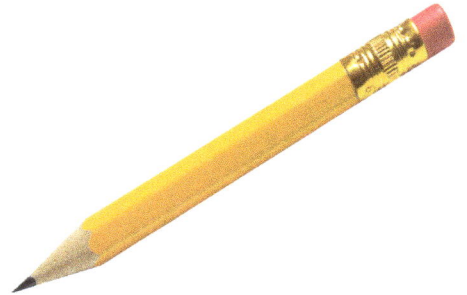 pencil
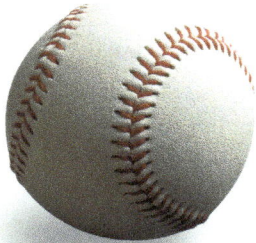 baseball	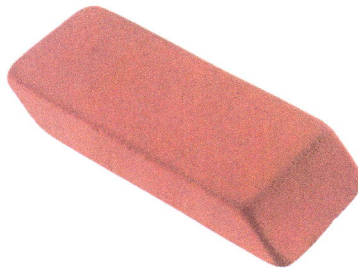 eraser	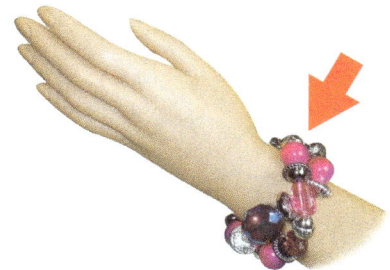 bracelet
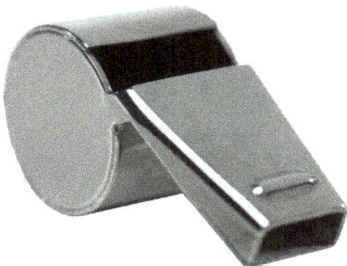 whistle	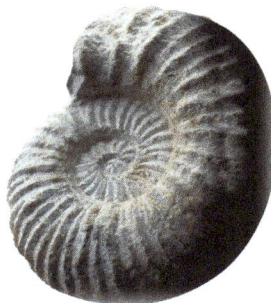 fossil	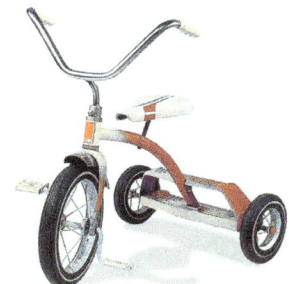 tricycle

Name _____

Helper Signature _____

Speech - Language Pathologist _____

Date _____

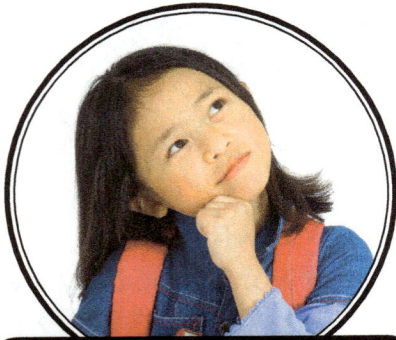

Jessie

This is Jessie. She was chasing all the things on this page.

S – Medial Position

1. Practice your sound by saying the words on this page. (Ex. bicycle, tassel, etc.). Say the last word twice.

2. Practice saying **Jessie** with each of the words. (Ex. Jessie bicycle, Jessie tassel, etc.). Say the last word pair twice.

3. Practice saying **was chasing** with these words. (Ex. Jessie was chasing a bicycle, etc.). Say one of the sentences twice.

4. Practice saying **classy** with these words. (Jessie was chasing a classy bicycle, etc.). Say one of the expanded sentences twice.

When you have finished this whole page you will have said your sound in 100 words! Good job!

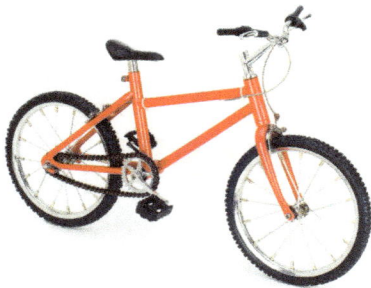 bicycle	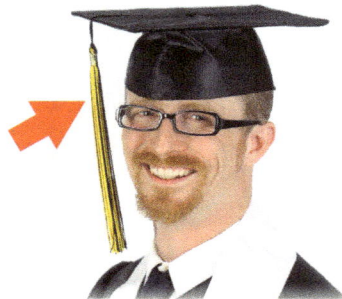 tassel	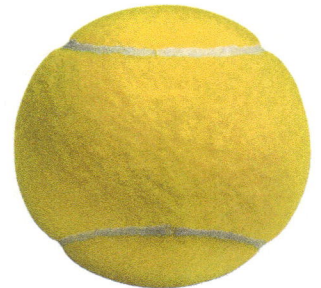 tennis ball
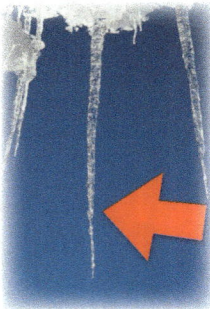 icicle	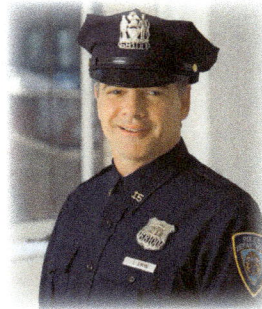 policeman	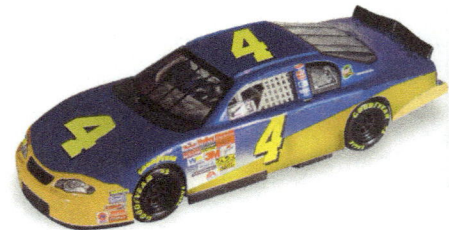 race car
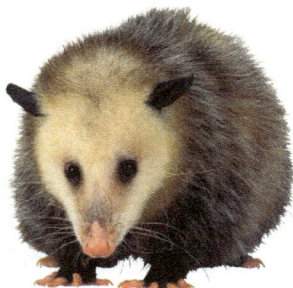 possum	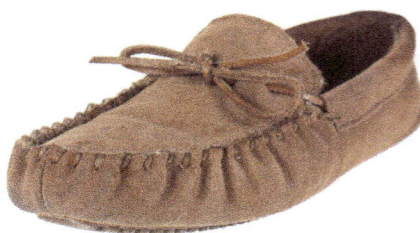 moccasin	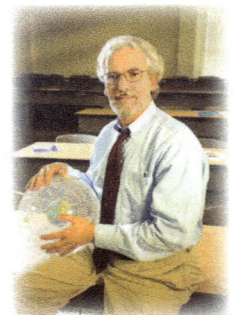 professor

Name _____

Speech - Language Pathologist _____

Helper Signature _____

Date _____

#BKCD-273 • *Say & Do® Artic Reps* • ©2015 Super Duper® Publications • www.superduperinc.com

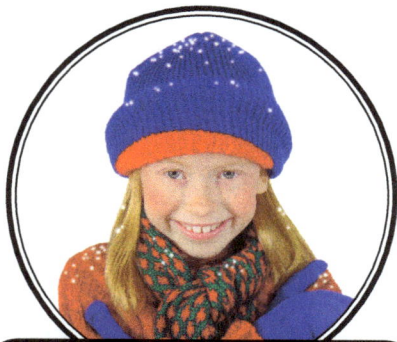

Cass

This is Cass. She makes all the things on this page.

1. Practice your sound by saying the words on this page. (Ex. vase, ace, etc.). Say the last word twice.

2. Practice saying **Cass** with each of the words. (Ex. Cass vase, Cass ace, etc.). Say the last word pair twice.

3. Practice saying **makes** with these words. (Ex. Cass makes a vase, etc.). Say one of the sentences twice.

4. Practice saying **brass** with these words. (Cass makes a brass vase, etc.). Say one of the expanded sentences twice.

When you have finished this whole page you will have said your sound in 100 words! Good job!

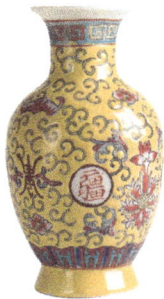 vase	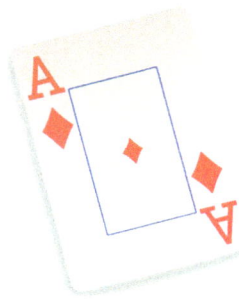 ace	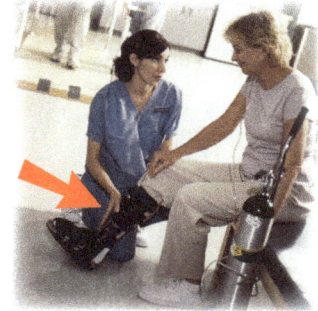 brace
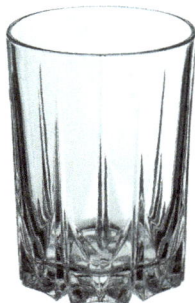 glass	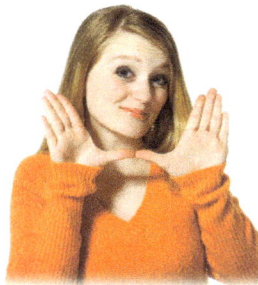 face	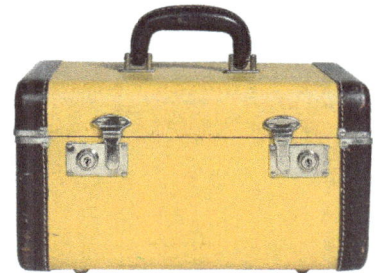 case
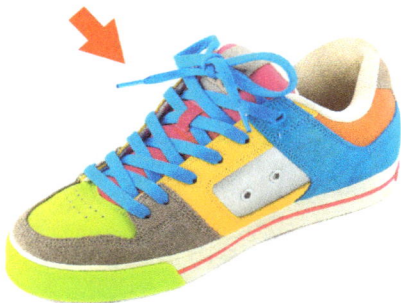 lace	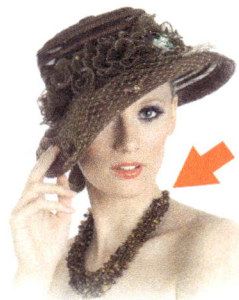 necklace	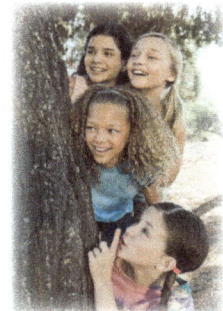 hiding place

Name _____

Helper Signature _____

Speech - Language Pathologist _____

Date _____

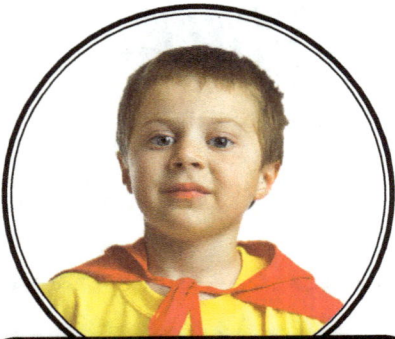

Wes

This is Wes. He takes all the things on this page.

1. Practice your sound by saying the words on this page. (Ex. piece, thermos, etc.). Say the last word twice.

2. Practice saying **Wes** with each of the words. (Ex. Wes piece, Wes thermos, etc.). Say the last word pair twice.

3. Practice saying **takes** with these words. (Ex. Wes takes a piece, etc.). Say one of the sentences twice.

4. Practice saying **enormous** with these words. (Wes takes an enormous piece, etc.). Say one of the expanded sentences twice.

When you have finished this whole page you will have said your sound in 100 words! Good job!

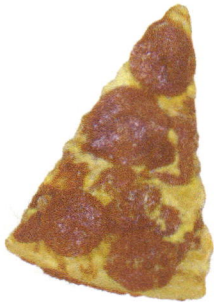 piece	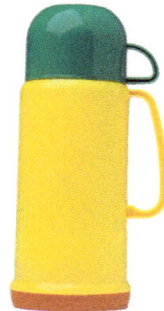 thermos	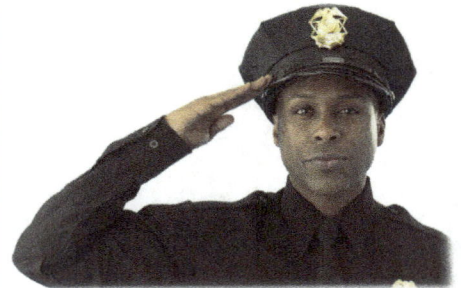 police
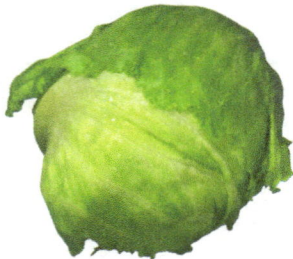 lettuce	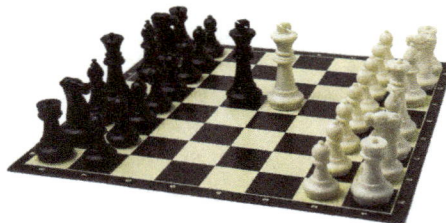 chess	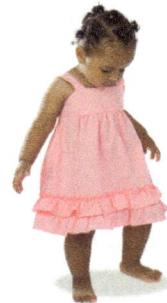 dress
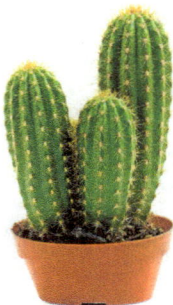 cactus	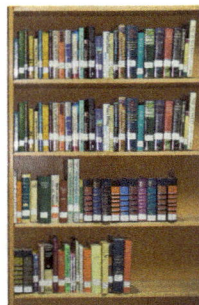 bookcase	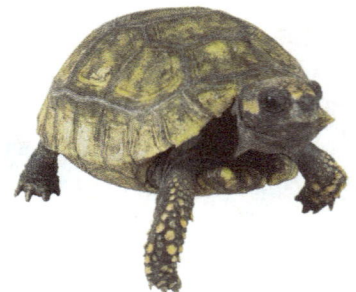 tortoise

Name _____

Helper Signature _____

Speech - Language Pathologist _____

Date _____

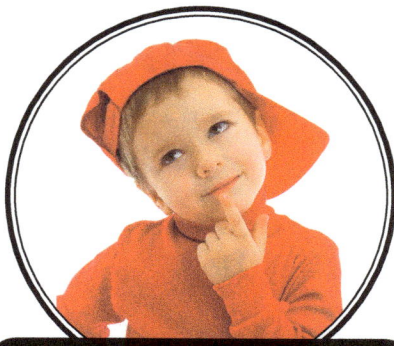

Chris

This is Chris. He picks all the things on this page.

S – Final Position

1. Practice your sound by saying the words on this page. (Ex. caboose, price, etc.). Say the last word twice.

2. Practice saying **Chris** with each of the words. (Ex. Chris caboose, Chris price, etc.). Say the last word pair twice.

3. Practice saying **picks** with these words. (Ex. Chris picks the caboose, etc.). Say one of the sentences twice.

4. Practice saying **nice** with these words. (Chris picks the nice caboose, etc.). Say one of the expanded sentences twice.

When you have finished this whole page you will have said your sound in 100 words! Good job!

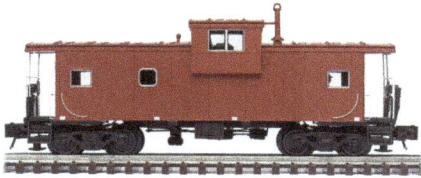

caboose

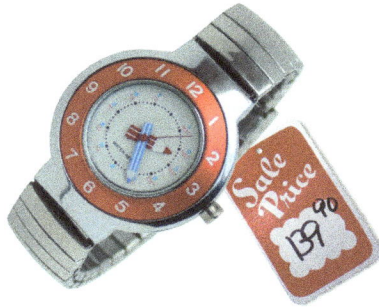

price

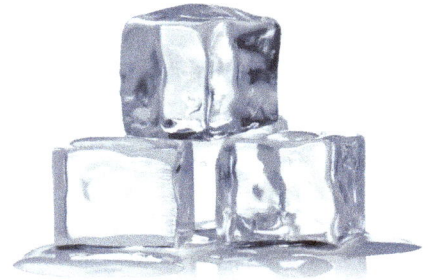

ice

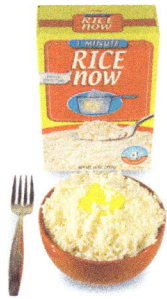

rice

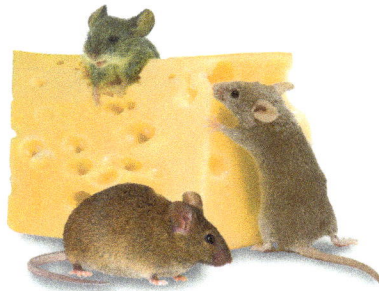

mice

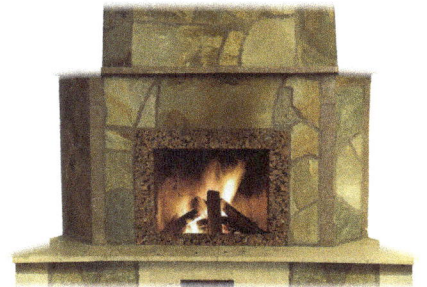

fireplace

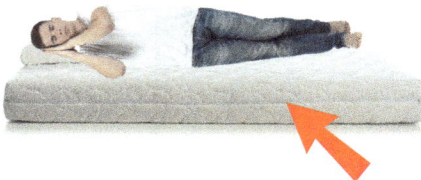

mattress

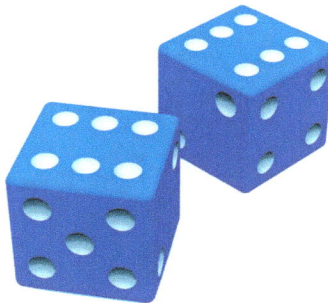

dice

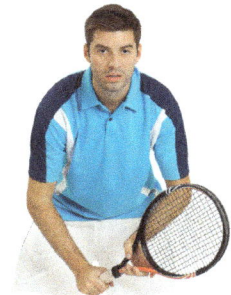

tennis

Name

Helper Signature

Speech - Language Pathologist

Date

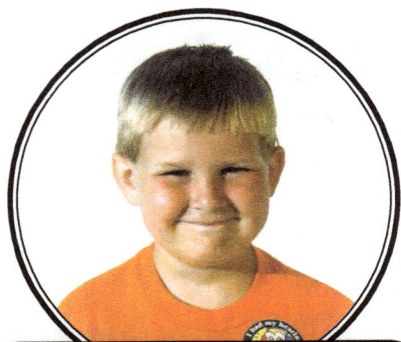

Gus

This is Gus. He looks at all the things on this page.

S – Final Position

1. Practice your sound by saying the words on this page. (Ex. bus, mouse, etc.). Say the last word twice.

2. Practice saying **Gus** with each of the words. (Ex. Gus bus, Gus mouse, etc.). Say the last word pair twice.

3. Practice saying **looks at** with these words. (Ex. Gus looks at the bus, etc.). Say one of the sentences twice.

4. Practice saying **famous** with these words. (Gus looks at a famous bus, etc.). Say one of the expanded sentences twice.

When you have finished this whole page you will have said your sound in 100 words! Good job!

bus	mouse	juice
blouse	octopus	Mother Goose
horse	floss	birdhouse

Name _____

Helper Signature _____

Speech - Language Pathologist _____

Date _____

#BKCD-273 • *Say & Do® Artic Reps* • ©2015 Super Duper® Publications • www.superduperinc.com

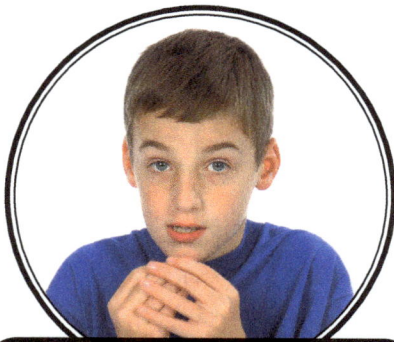

Scotty

This is Scotty. He scared all the things on this page.

SK – Blend

1. Practice your sound by saying the words on this page. (Ex. scarecrow, school bus, etc.). Say the last word twice.

2. Practice saying **Scotty** with each of the words. (Ex. Scotty scarecrow, Scotty school bus, etc.). Say the last word pair twice.

3. Practice saying **scared** with these words. (Ex. Scotty scared a scarecrow, etc.). Say one of the sentences twice.

4. Practice saying **squeaky** with these words. (Scotty scared a squeaky scarecrow, etc.). Say one of the expanded sentences twice.

When you have finished this whole page you will have said your sound in 100 words! Good job!

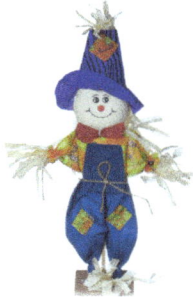 scarecrow	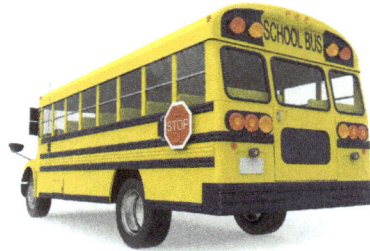 school bus	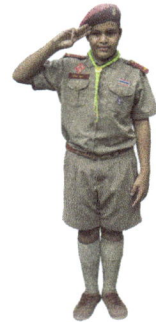 scout
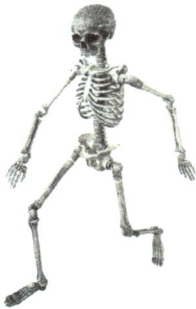 skeleton	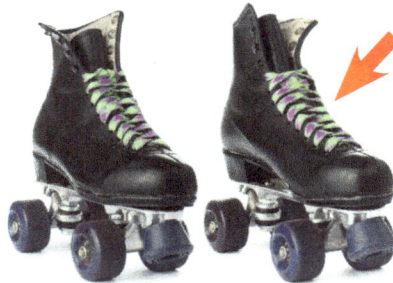 skate	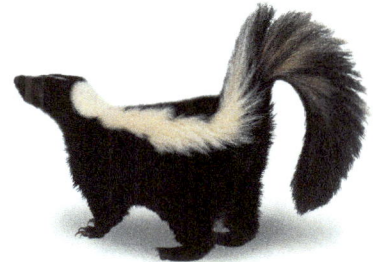 skunk
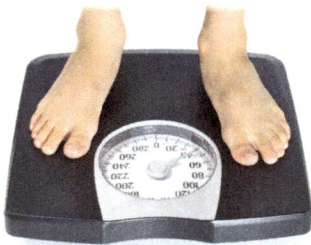 scale	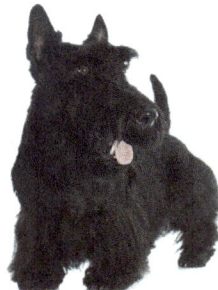 scottie	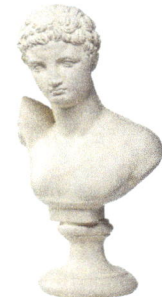 sculpture

Name _____

Helper Signature _____

Speech - Language Pathologist _____

Date _____

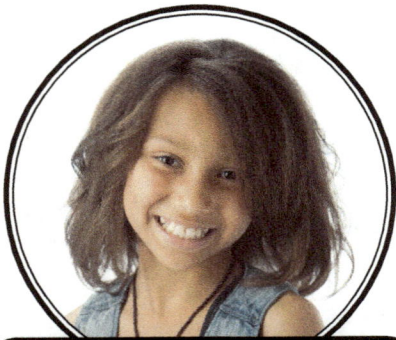

Scarlett

This is Scarlett. She sketched all the things on this page.

1. Practice your sound by saying the words on this page. (Ex. skier, school, etc.). Say the last word twice.

2. Practice saying **Scarlett** with each of the words. (Ex. Scarlett skier, Scarlett school, etc.). Say the last word pair twice.

3. Practice saying **sketched** with these words. (Ex. Scarlett sketched a skier, etc.). Say one of the sentences twice.

4. Practice saying **skilled** with these words. (Scarlett sketched a skilled skier, etc.). Say one of the expanded sentences twice.

When you have finished this whole page you will have said your sound in 100 words! Good job!

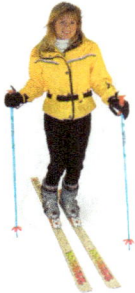 skier	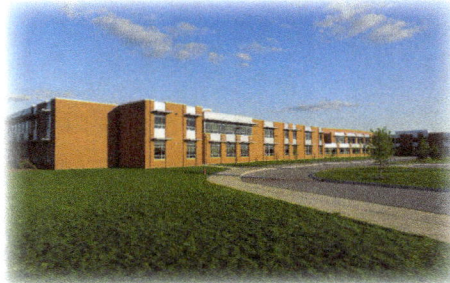 school	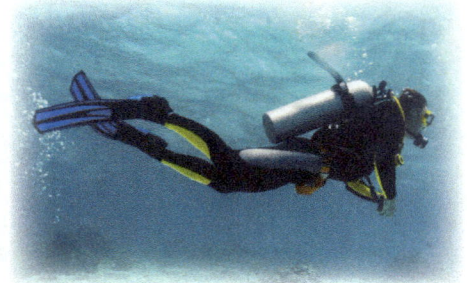 scuba diver
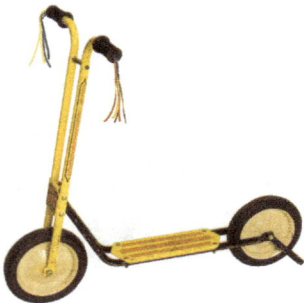 scooter	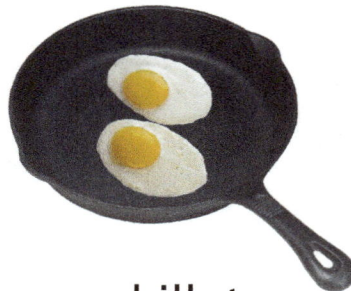 skillet	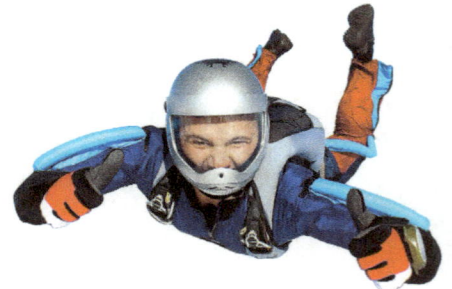 skydiver
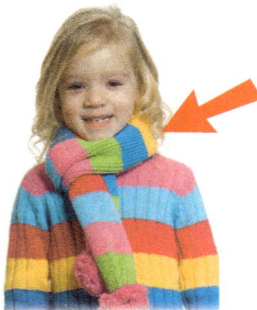 scarf	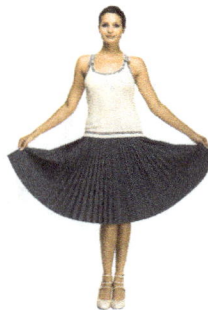 skirt	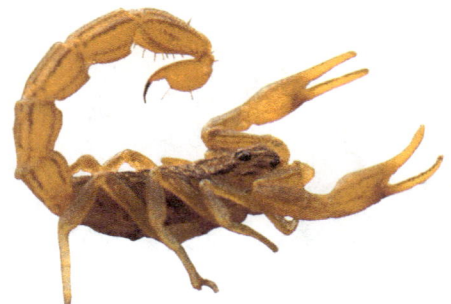 scorpion

Name _____

Helper Signature _____

Speech - Language Pathologist _____

Date _____

#BKCD-273 • *Say & Do® Artic Reps* • ©2015 Super Duper® Publications • www.superduperinc.com

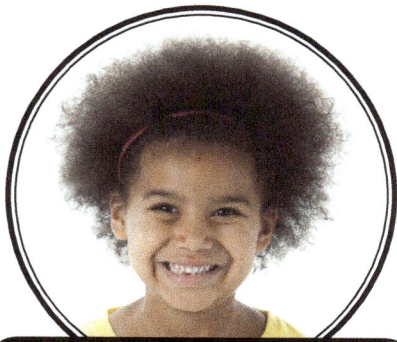

Josslyn

This is Josslyn. She slipped on all the things on this page.

1. Practice your sound by saying the words on this page. (Ex. slingshot, cole slaw, etc.). Say the last word twice.

2. Practice saying **Josslyn** with each of the words. (Ex. Josslyn slingshot, Josslyn cole slaw, etc.). Say the last word pair twice.

3. Practice saying **slipped on** with these words. (Ex. Josslyn slipped on the slingshot, etc.). Say one of the sentences twice.

4. Practice saying **slick** with these words. (Josslyn slipped on a slick slingshot, etc.). Say one of the expanded sentences twice.

When you have finished this whole page you will have said your sound in 100 words! Good job!

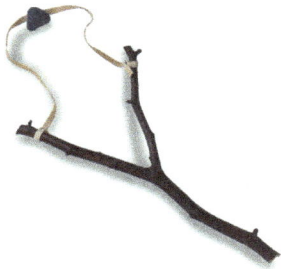 slingshot	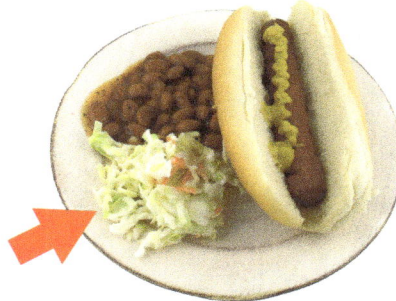 cole slaw	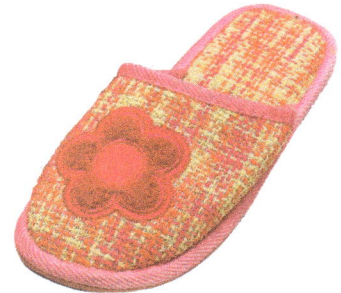 slipper
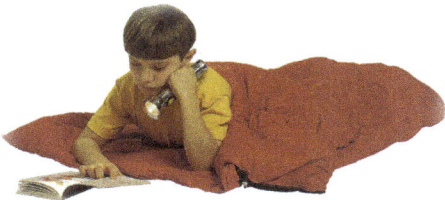 sleeping bag	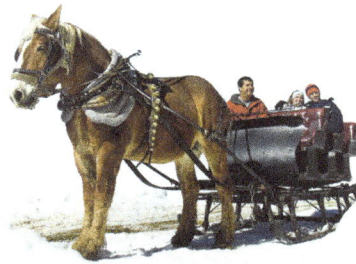 sleigh	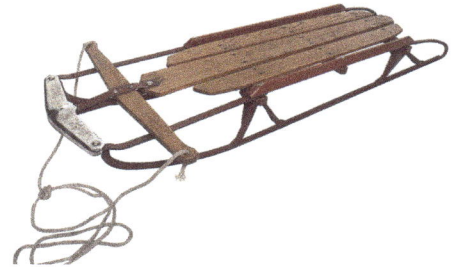 sled
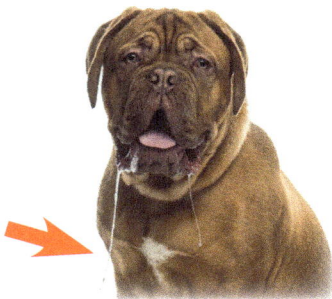 slobber	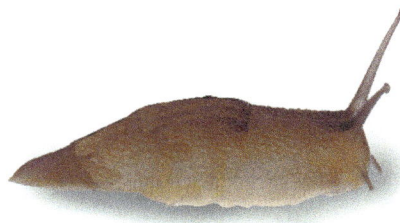 slug	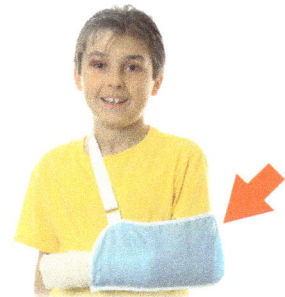 sling

Name _____

Helper Signature _____

Speech - Language Pathologist _____

Date _____

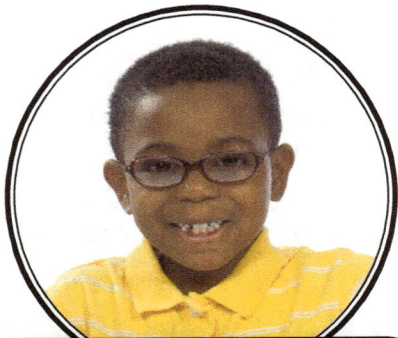

Wesley

This is Wesley. He sleeps on all the things on this page.

1. Practice your sound by saying the words on this page. (Ex. slide, dog sled, etc.). Say the last word twice.

2. Practice saying **Wesley** with each of the words. (Ex. Wesley slide, Wesley dog sled, etc.). Say the last word pair twice.

3. Practice saying **sleeps on** with these words. (Ex. Wesley sleeps on the slide, etc.). Say one of the sentences twice.

4. Practice saying **slim** with these words. (Wesley sleeps on the slim slide, etc.). Say one of the expanded sentences twice.

When you have finished this whole page you will have said your sound in 100 words! Good job!

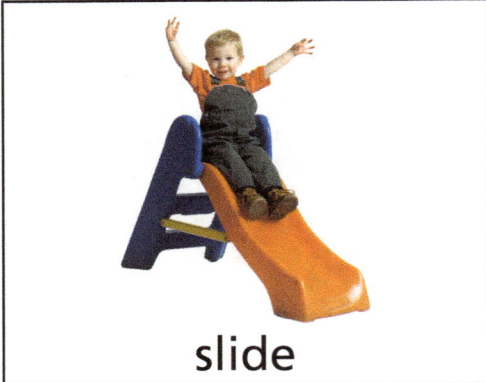
slide

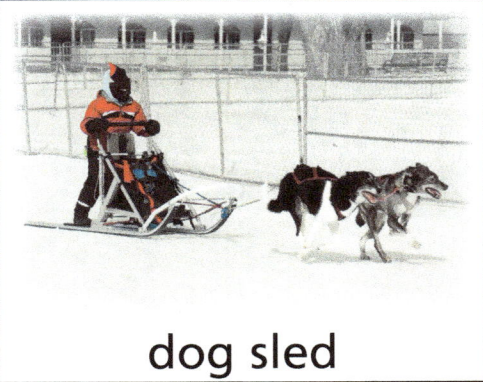
dog sled

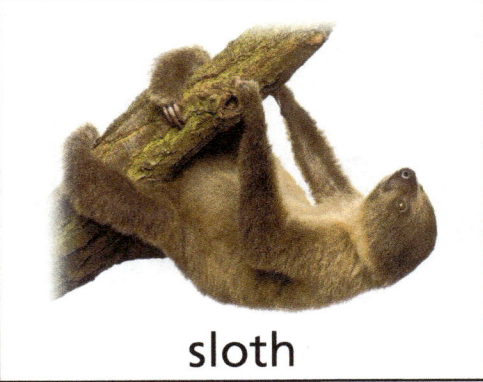
sloth

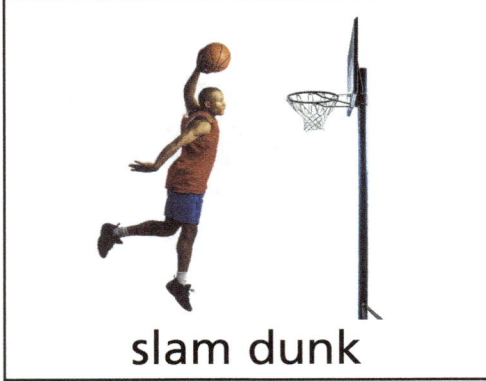
slam dunk

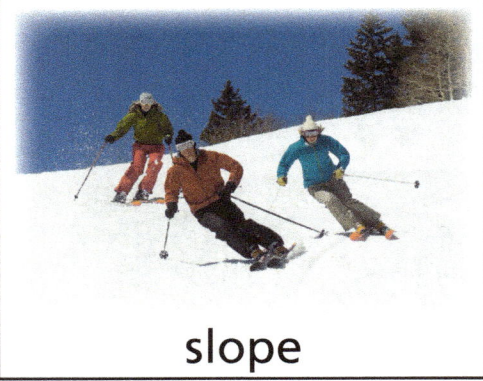
slope

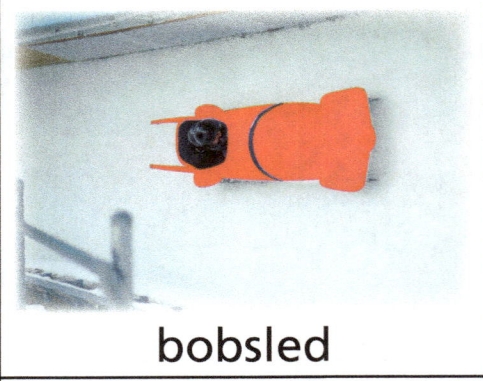
bobsled

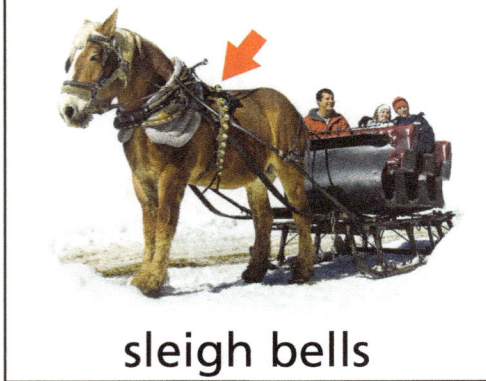
sleigh bells

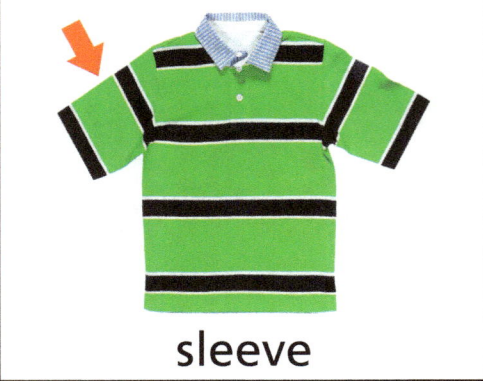
sleeve

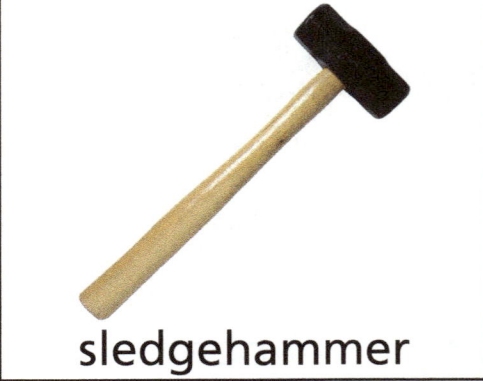
sledgehammer

Name _____

Helper Signature _____

Speech - Language Pathologist _____

Date _____

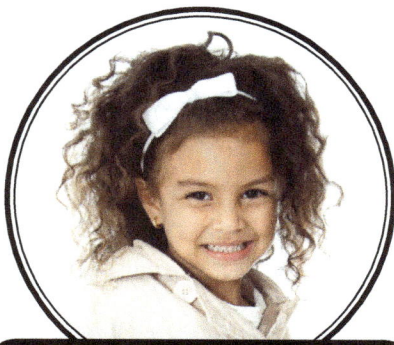

Smilla

This is Smilla. She smiles at all the things on this page.

1. Practice your sound by saying the words on this page. (Ex. blacksmith, smog, etc.). Say the last word twice.
2. Practice saying **Smilla** with each of the words. (Ex. Smilla blacksmith, Smilla smog, etc.). Say the last word pair twice.
3. Practice saying **smiles at** with these words. (Ex. Smilla smiles at the blacksmith, etc.). Say one of the sentences twice.
4. Practice saying **smart** with these words. (Smilla smiles at the smart blacksmith, etc.). Say one of the expanded sentences twice.

When you have finished this whole page you will have said your sound in 100 words! Good job!

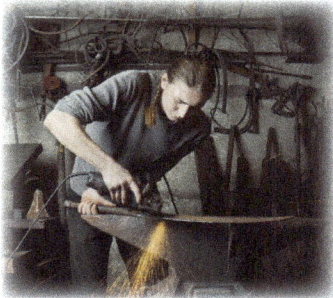
blacksmith

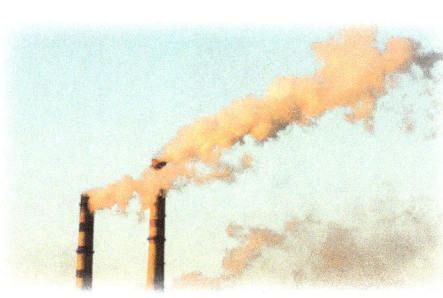
smog

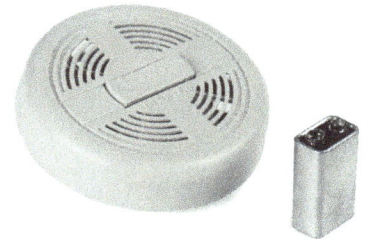
smoke detector

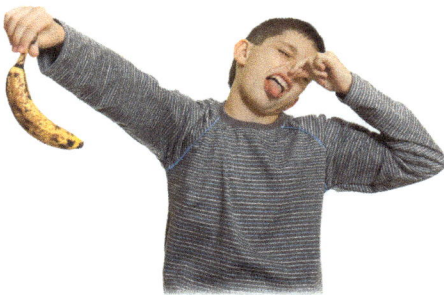
smelly banana

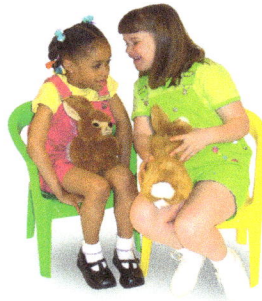
small talk

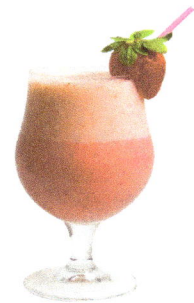
smoothie

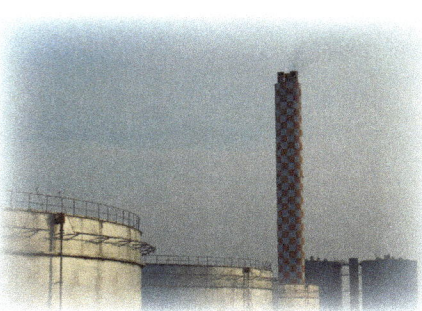
smokestack

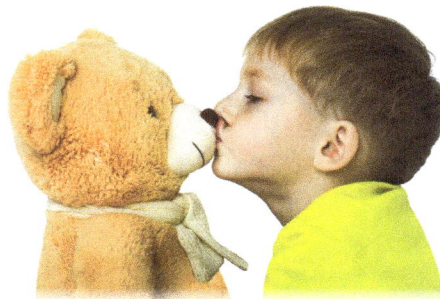
smooch

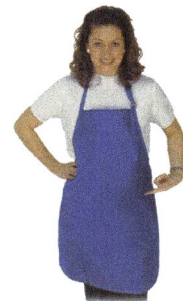
smock

Name _____

Helper Signature _____

Speech - Language Pathologist _____

Date _____

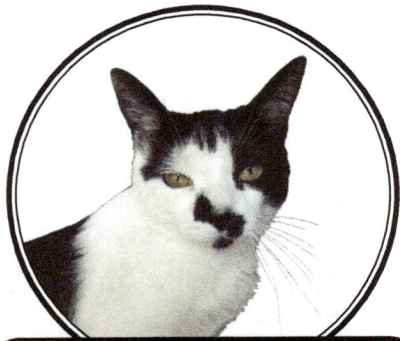

Smitty

This is Smitty. He smelled all the things on this page.

SM – Blends

1. Practice your sound by saying the words on this page. (Ex. smoke, smart graduate, etc.). Say the last word twice.

2. Practice saying **Smitty** with each of the words. (Ex. Smitty smoke, Smitty smart graduate, etc.). Say the last word pair twice.

3. Practice saying **smelled** with these words. (Ex. Smitty smelled smoke, etc.). Say one of the sentences twice.

4. Practice saying **small** with these words. (Smitty smelled small smoke, etc.). Say one of the expanded sentences twice.

When you have finished this whole page you will have said your sound in 100 words! Good job!

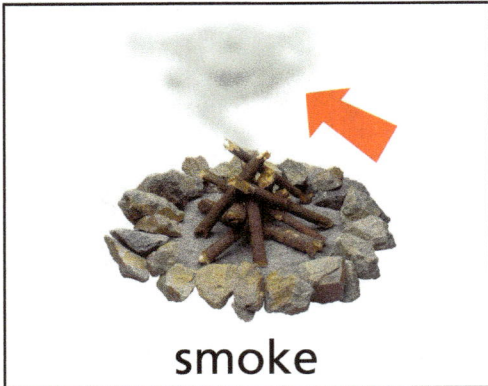 smoke	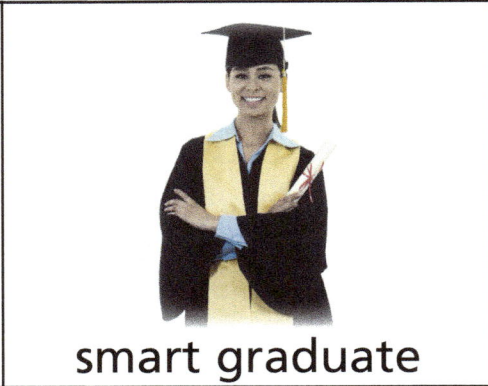 smart graduate	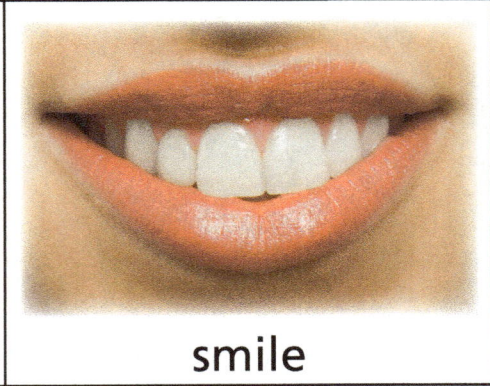 smile
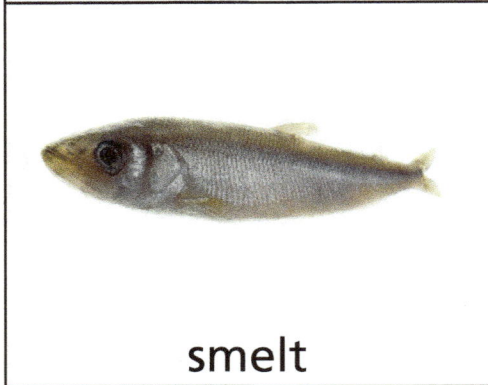 smelt	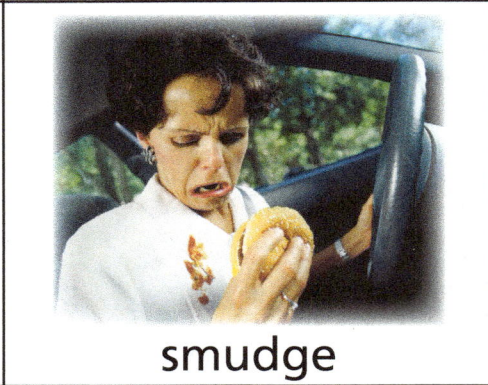 smudge	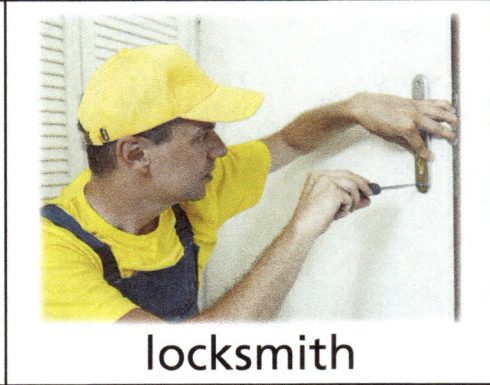 locksmith
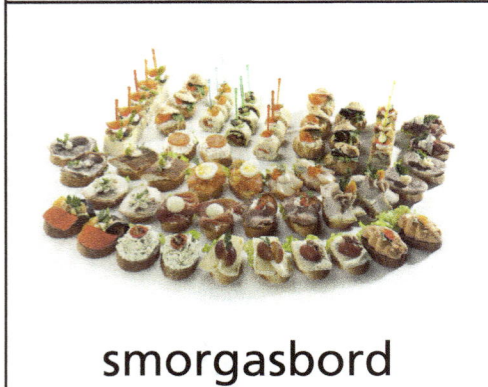 smorgasbord	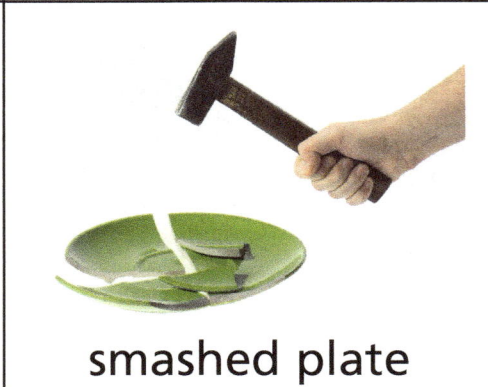 smashed plate	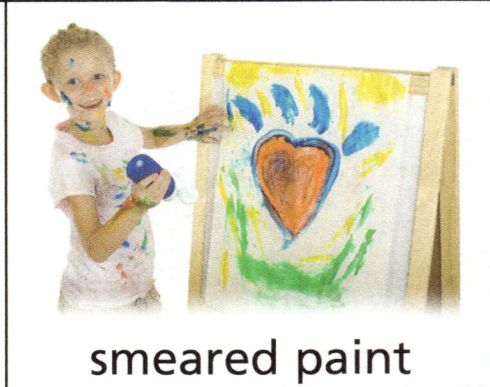 smeared paint

Name

Helper Signature

Speech - Language Pathologist

Date

#BKCD-273 • *Say & Do® Artic Reps* • ©2015 Super Duper® Publications • www.superduperinc.com

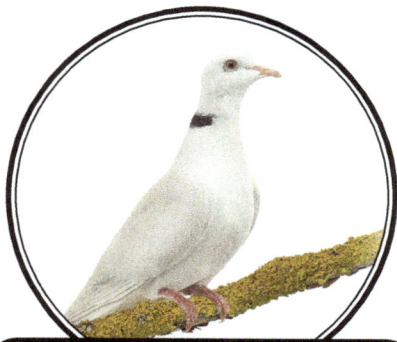

Snowy

This is Snowy. He snuggled with all the things on this page.

SN – Blend

1. Practice your sound by saying the words on this page. (Ex. snowman, snare drum, etc.). Say the last word twice.

2. Practice saying **Snowy** with each of the words. (Ex. Snowy snowman, Snowy snare drum, etc.). Say the last word pair twice.

3. Practice saying **snuggled with** these words. (Ex. Snowy snuggled with a snowman, etc.). Say one of the sentences twice.

4. Practice saying **snazzy** with these words. (Snowy snuggled with a snazzy snowman etc.). Say one of the expanded sentences twice.

When you have finished this whole page you will have said your sound in 100 words! Good job!

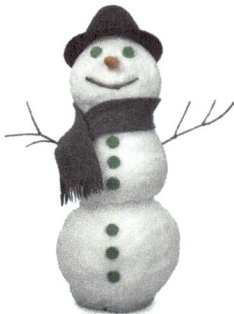 snowman	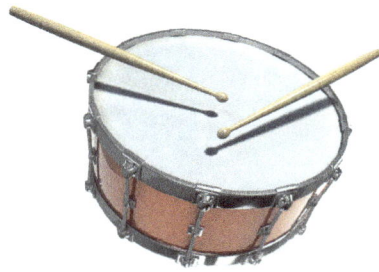 snare drum	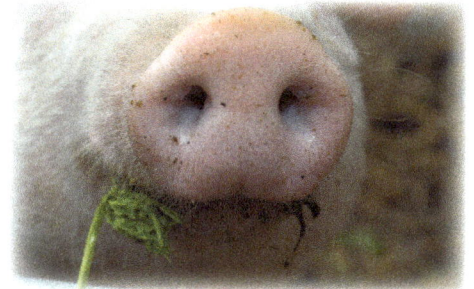 snout
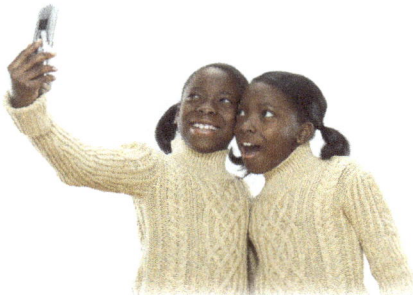 snapshot	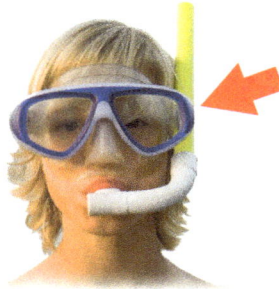 snorkel	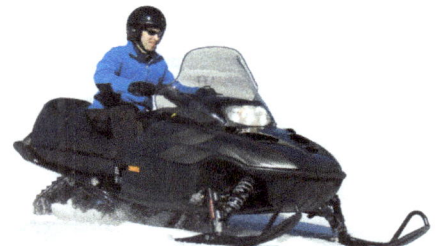 snowmobile
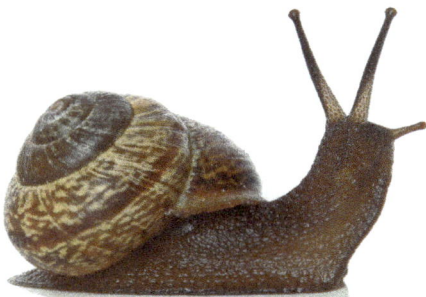 snail	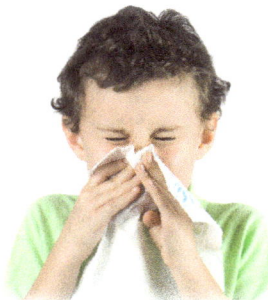 sneeze	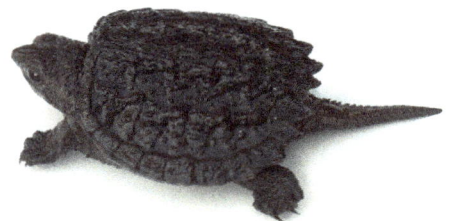 snapping turtle

Name

Speech - Language Pathologist

Helper Signature

Date

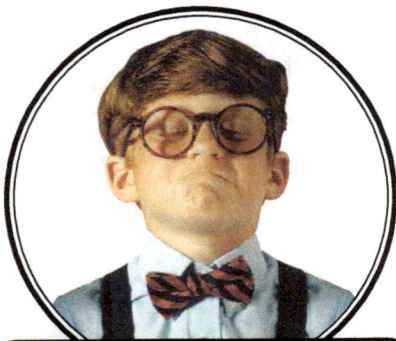

Snyder

This is Snyder. He sniffed all the things on this page.

1. Practice your sound by saying the words on this page. (Ex. snacks, snap dragon, etc.). Say the last word twice.

2. Practice saying **Snyder** with each of the words. (Ex. Snyder snacks, Snyder snap dragon, etc.). Say the last word pair twice.

3. Practice saying **sniffed** with these words. (Ex. Snyder sniffed the snacks, etc.). Say one of the sentences twice.

4. Practice saying **snobby** with these words. (Snyder sniffed the snobby snacks etc.). Say one of the expanded sentences twice.

When you have finished this whole page you will have said your sound in 100 words! Good job!

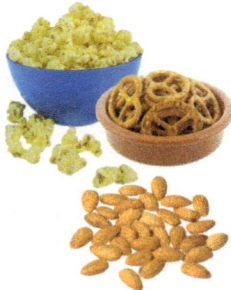 snacks	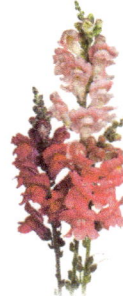 snap dragon	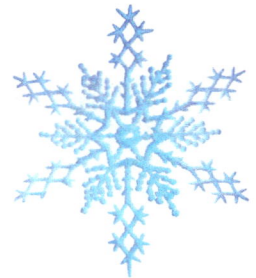 snowflake
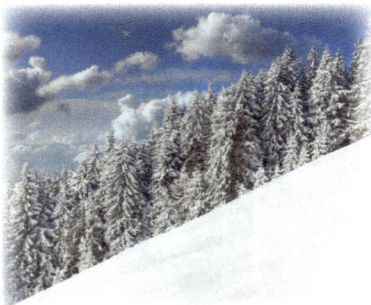 snow	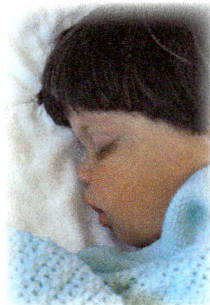 snoring child	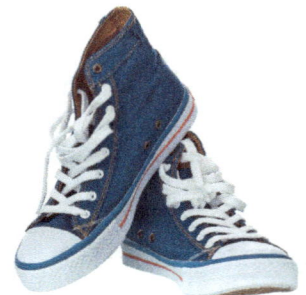 sneakers
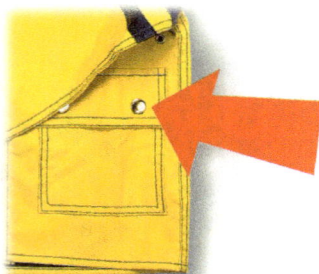 snap	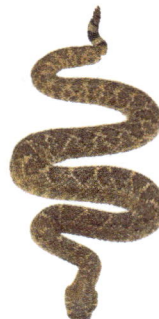 snake	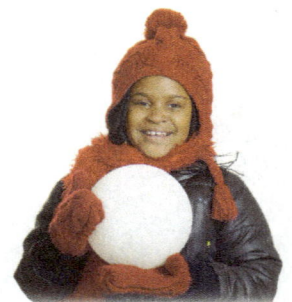 snowball

Name

Speech - Language Pathologist

Helper Signature

Date

#BKCD-273 • *Say & Do*® Artic Reps •©2015 Super Duper® Publications • www.superduperinc.com

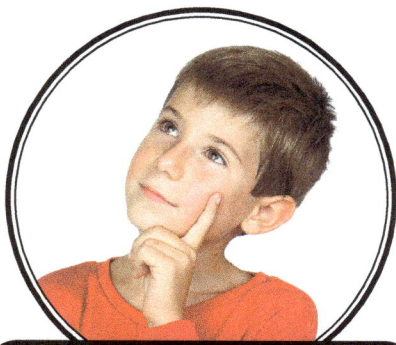

Spencer

This is Spencer. He spotted all the things on this page.

SP – Blend

1. Practice your sound by saying the words on this page. (Ex. spice, sports, etc.). Say the last word twice.

2. Practice saying **Spencer** with each of the words. (Ex. Spencer spice, Spencer sports, etc.). Say the last word pair twice.

3. Practice saying **spotted** with these words. (Ex. Spencer spotted a spice, etc.). Say one of the sentences twice.

4. Practice saying **speckled** with these words. (Spencer spotted the speckled spice, etc.). Say one of the expanded sentences twice.

   When you have finished this whole page you will have said your sound in 100 words! Good job!

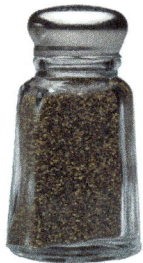 spice	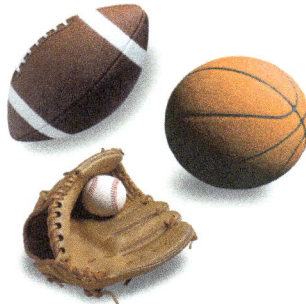 sports	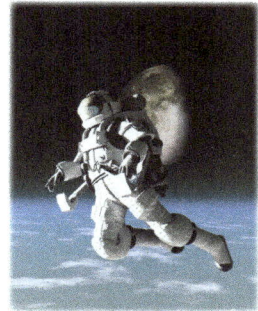 space
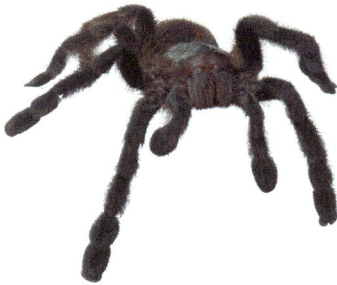 spider	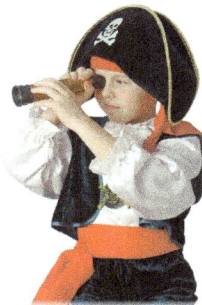 spy	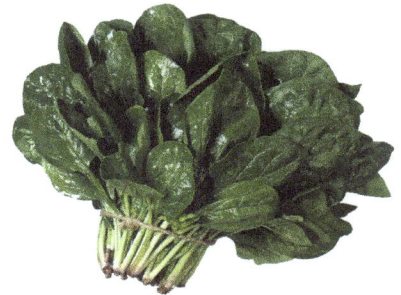 spinach
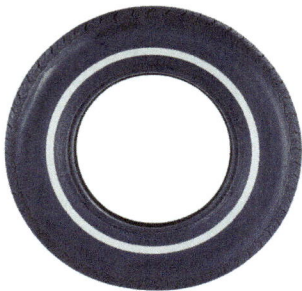 spare tire	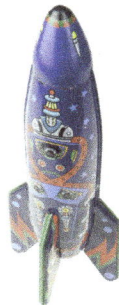 spaceship	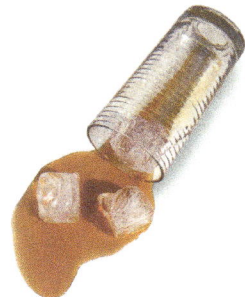 spilled tea

Name _____

Helper Signature _____

Speech - Language Pathologist _____

Date _____

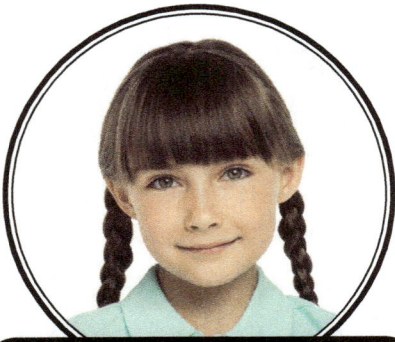

Sparrow

This is Sparrow. She spins all the things on this page.

1. Practice your sound by saying the words on this page. (Ex. speakers, spider web, etc.). Say the last word twice.

2. Practice saying **Sparrow** with each of the words. (Ex. Sparrow speakers, Sparrow spider web, etc.). Say the last word pair twice.

3. Practice saying **spins** with these words. (Ex. Sparrow spins speakers, etc.). Say one of the sentences twice.

4. Practice saying **special** with these words. (Sparrow spins special speakers, etc.). Say one of the expanded sentences twice.

When you have finished this whole page you will have said your sound in 100 words! Good job!

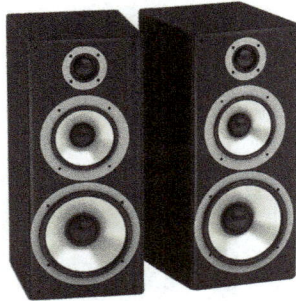
speakers

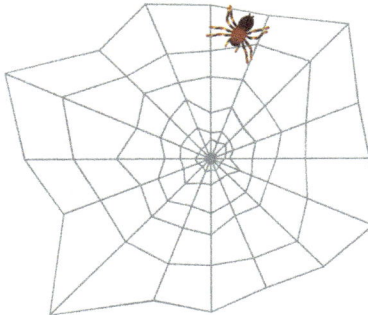
spider web

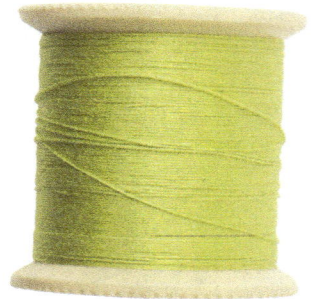
spool

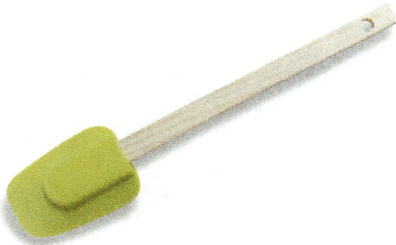
spatula

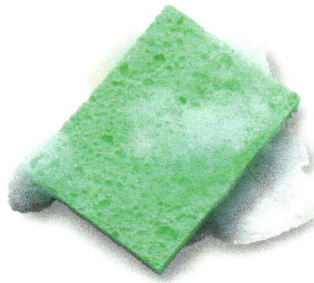
sponge

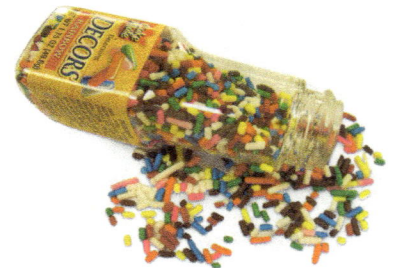
sprinkles

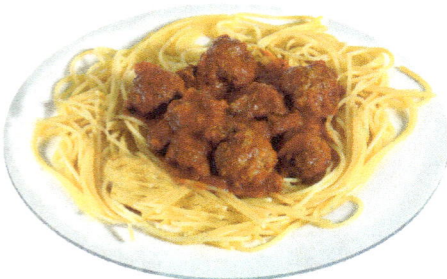
spaghetti

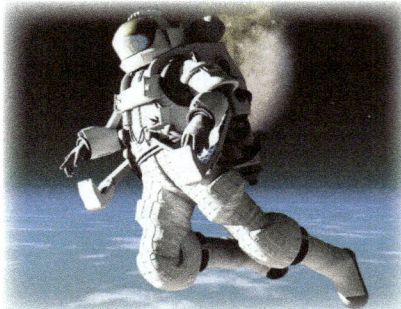
space suit

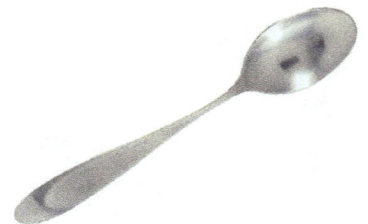
spoon

Name _____

Helper Signature _____

Speech - Language Pathologist _____

Date _____

#BKCD-273 • *Say & Do® Artic Reps* • ©2015 Super Duper® Publications • www.superduperinc.com

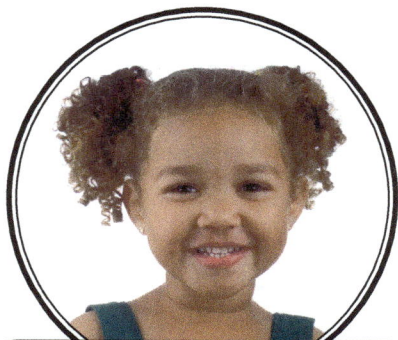

Stella

This is Stella. She stacks all the things on this page.

ST – Blend

1. Practice your sound by saying the words on this page. (Ex. stamps, stork, etc.). Say the last word twice.

2. Practice saying **Stella** with each of the words. (Ex. Stella stamps, Stella stork, etc.). Say the last word pair twice.

3. Practice saying **stacks** on with these words. (Ex. Stella stacks stamps, etc.). Say one of the sentences twice.

4. Practice saying **sticky** with these words. (Stella stacks sticky stamps, etc.). Say one of the expanded sentences twice.

When you have finished this whole page you will have said your sound in 100 words! Good job!

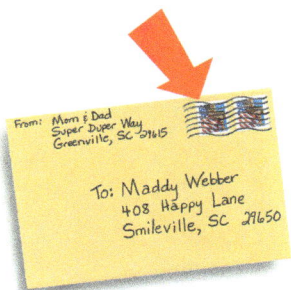 stamps	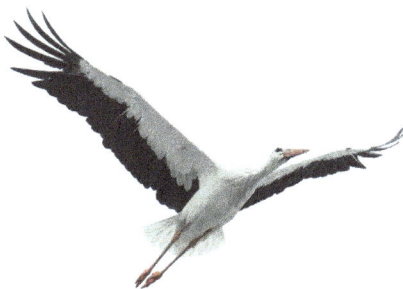 stork	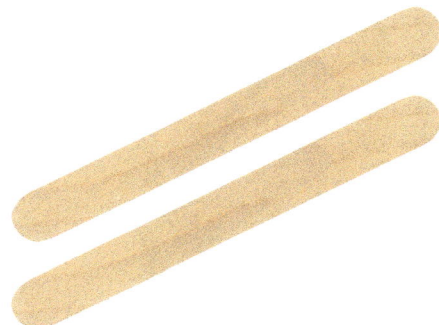 sticks
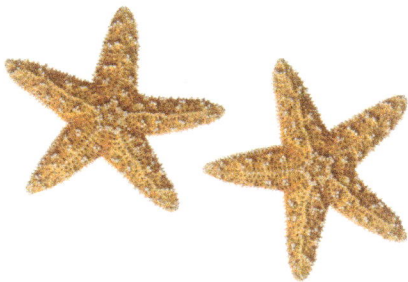 starfish	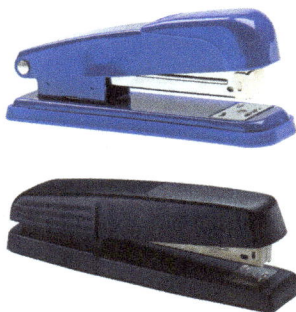 staplers	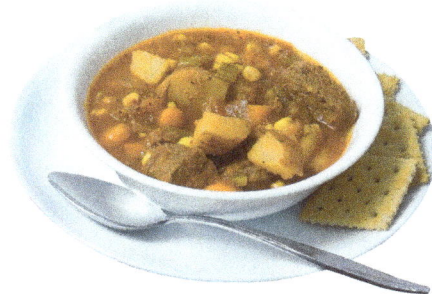 stew
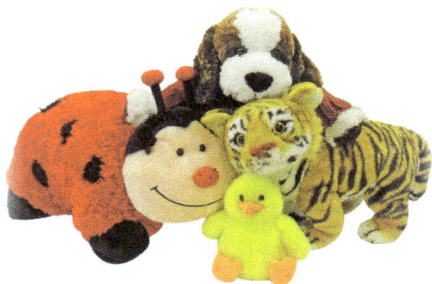 stuffed animals	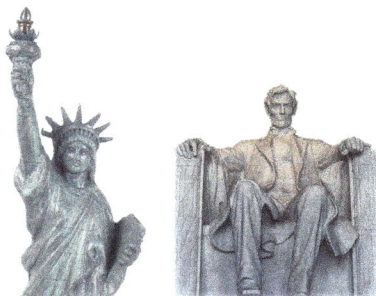 statues	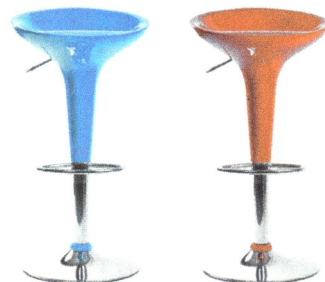 stools

Name _____

Helper Signature _____

Speech - Language Pathologist _____

Date _____

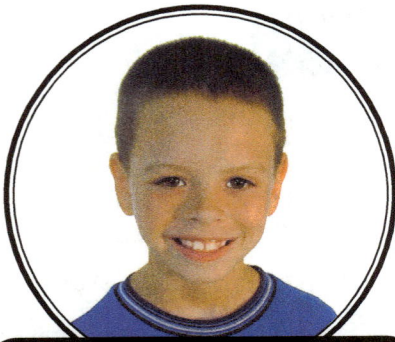

ST – Blend

Steve

This is Steve. He stumbled on all the things on this page.

1. Practice your sound by saying the words on this page. (Ex. stairs, stop sign, etc.). Say the last word twice.
2. Practice saying **Steve** with each of the words. (Ex. Steve stairs, Steve stop sign, etc.). Say the last word pair twice.
3. Practice saying **stumbled on** with these words. (Ex. Steve stumbled on stairs, etc.). Say one of the sentences twice.
4. Practice saying **stinky** with these words. (Steve stumbled on stinky stairs, etc.). Say one of the expanded sentences twice.

When you have finished this whole page you will have said your sound in 100 words! Good job!

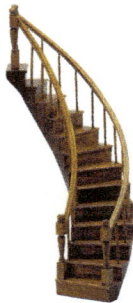 stairs	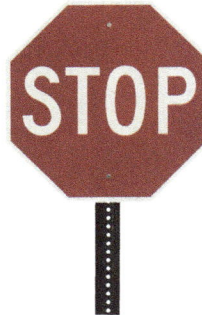 stop sign	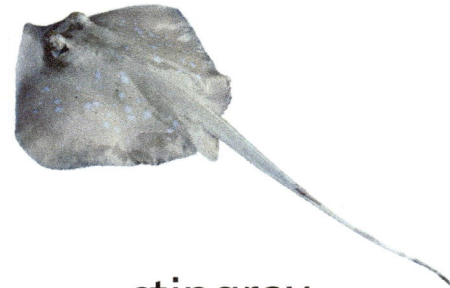 stingray
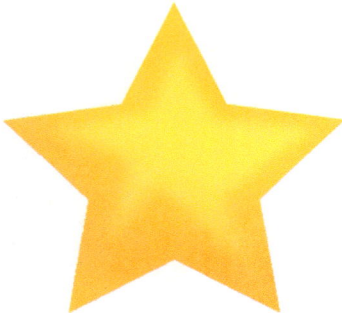 star	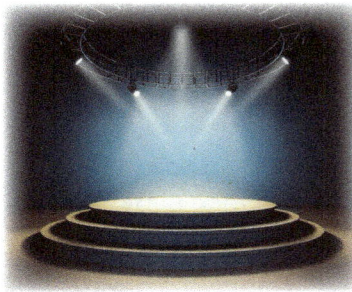 stage	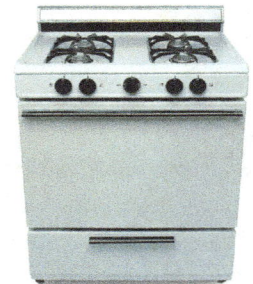 stove
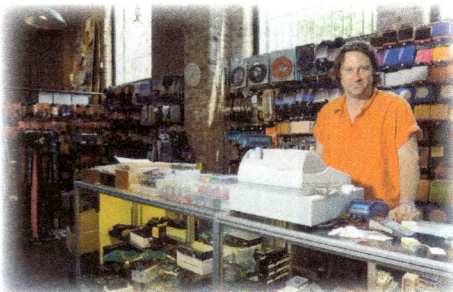 store	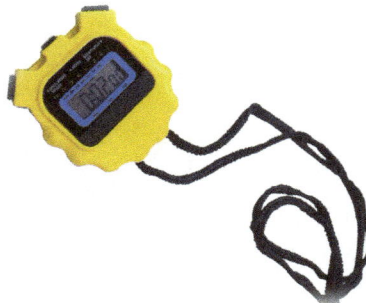 stopwatch	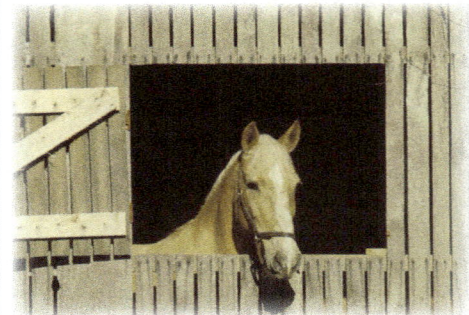 stable

Name _____

Helper Signature _____

Speech - Language Pathologist _____

Date _____

#BKCD-273 • *Say & Do® Artic Reps* • ©2015 Super Duper® Publications • www.superduperinc.com

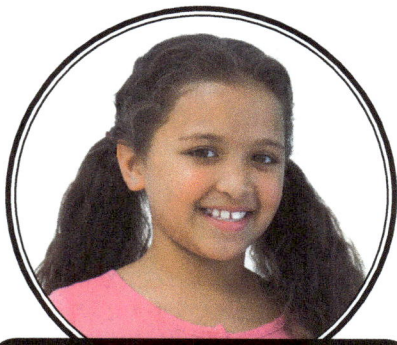

SW – Blend

1. Practice your sound by saying the words on this page. (Ex. fly swatter, swarm, etc.). Say the last word twice.

2. Practice saying **Swann** with each of the words. (Ex. Swann fly swatter, Swann swarm, etc.). Say the last word pair twice.

3. Practice saying **swirls** on with these words. (Ex. Swann swirls a fly swatter, etc.). Say one of the sentences twice.

4. Practice saying **sweet** with these words. (Swann swirls a sweet fly swatter, etc.). Say one of the expanded sentences twice.

When you have finished this whole page you will have said your sound in 100 words! Good job!

Swann

This is Swann. She swirls all the things on this page.

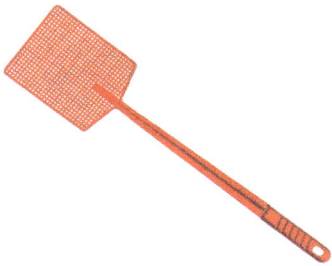

fly swatter

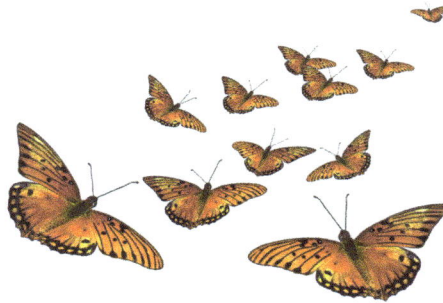

swarm

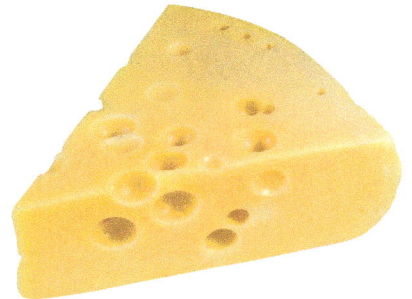

swiss cheese

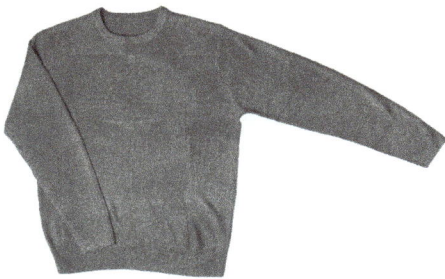

sweatshirt

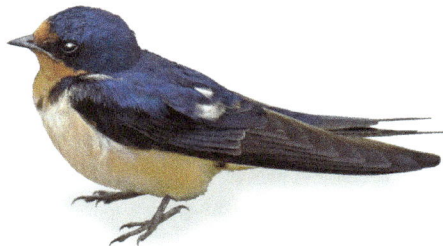

swallow

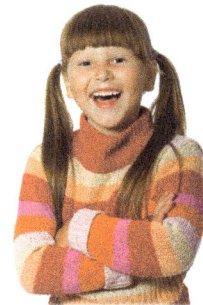

sweater

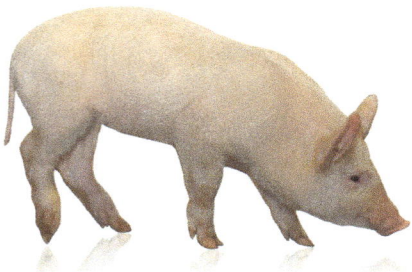

swine

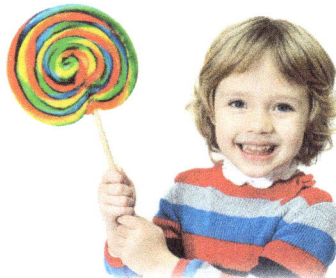

sweet treat

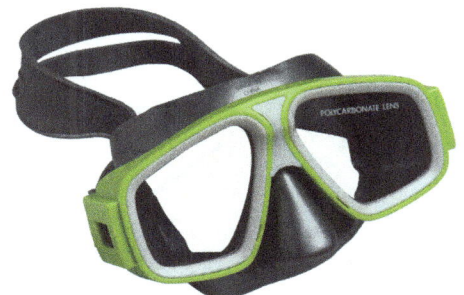

swim mask

Name _____

Helper Signature _____

Speech - Language Pathologist _____

Date _____

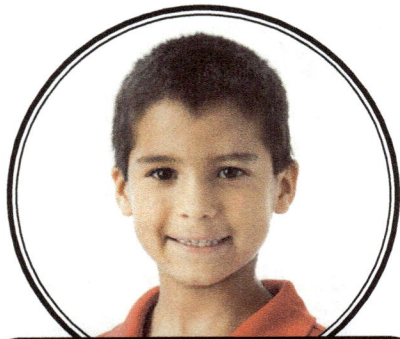

SW – Blend

Swensen

Swensen

This is Swensen. He swiped all the things on this page.

1. Practice your sound by saying the words on this page. (Ex. suede boots, swim fins, etc.). Say the last word twice.

2. Practice saying **Swensen** with each of the words. (Ex. Swensen suede boots, Swensen swim fins, etc.). Say the last word pair twice.

3. Practice saying **swiped** on with these words. (Ex. Swensen swiped suede boots, etc.). Say one of the sentences twice.

4. Practice saying **Swiss** with these words. (Swensen swiped Swiss suede boots, etc.). Say one of the expanded sentences twice.

When you have finished this whole page you will have said your sound in 100 words! Good job!

suede boots	swim fins	sweet peas
swing	sweat	swimsuit
swamp	swan	sweatpants

Name

Helper Signature

Speech - Language Pathologist

Date

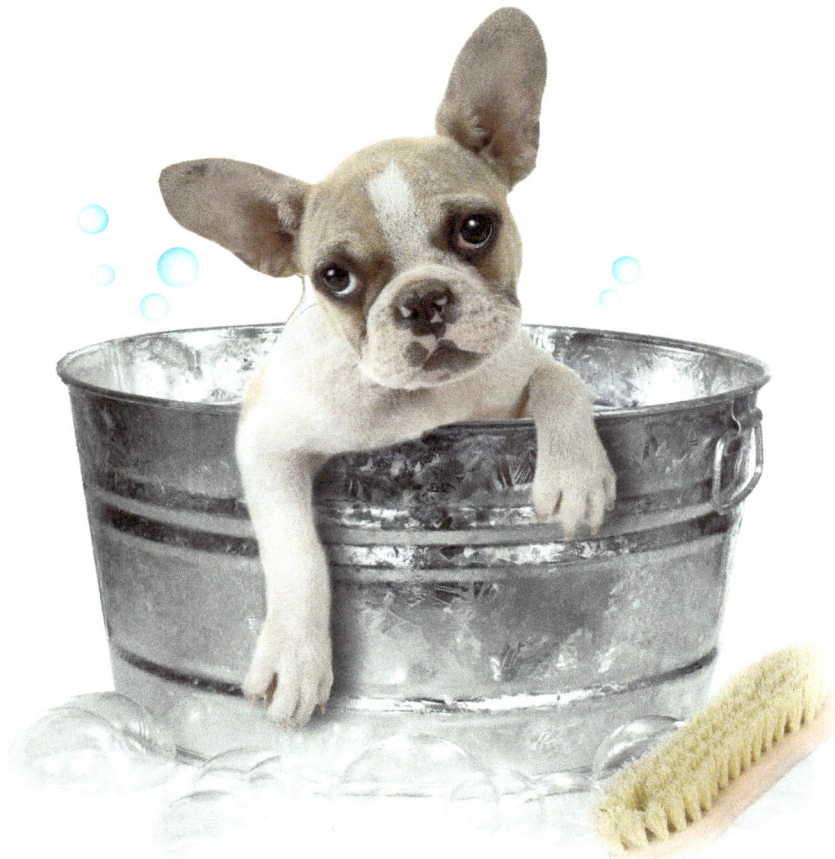

SH

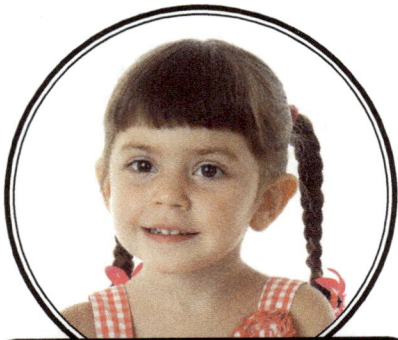

Shari

This is Shari. She shared all the things on this page.

1. Practice your sound by saying the words on this page. (Ex. shark, short child etc.). Say the last word twice.

2. Practice saying **Shari** with each of the words. (Ex. Shari shark, Shari short child, etc.). Say the last word pair twice.

3. Practice saying **shared** with these words. (Ex. Shari shared a shark, etc.). Say one of the sentences twice.

4. Practice saying **sharp** with these words. (Shari shared a sharp shark, etc.). Say one of the expanded sentences twice.

When you have finished this whole page you will have said your sound in 100 words! Good job!

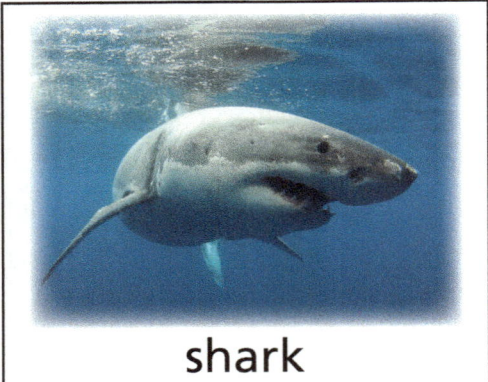 shark	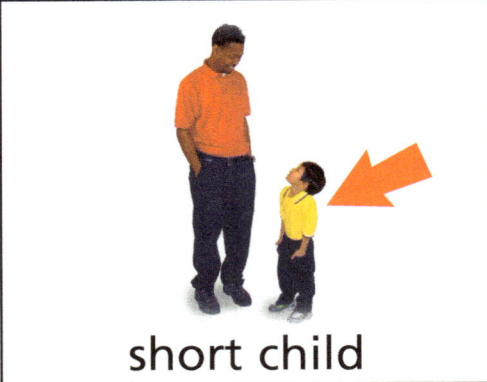 short child	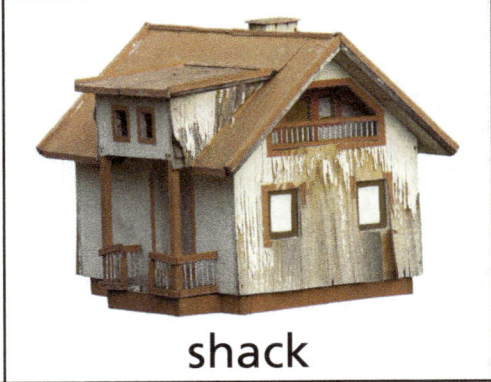 shack
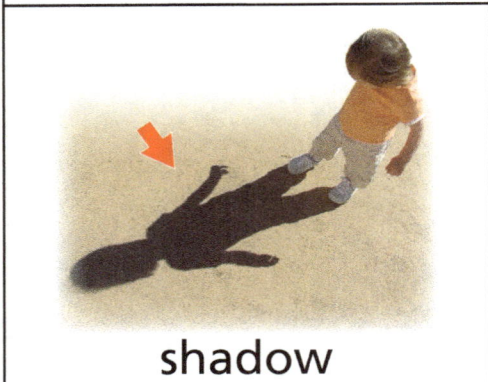 shadow	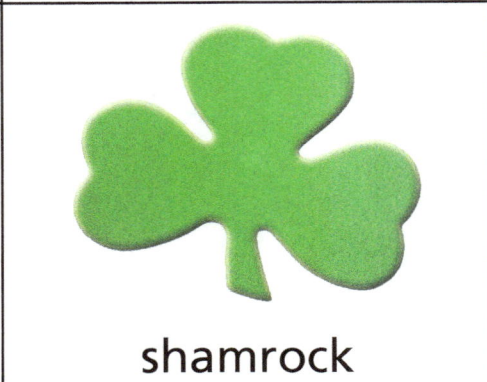 shamrock	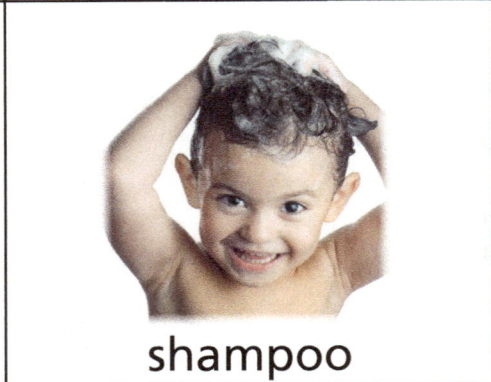 shampoo
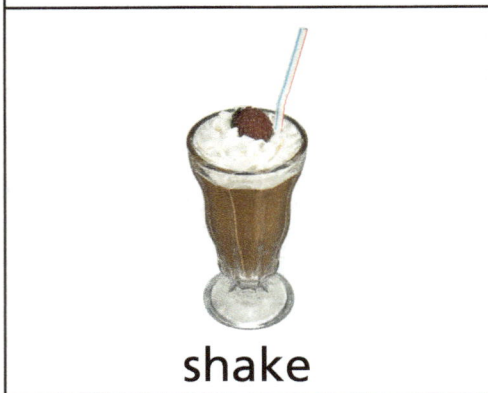 shake	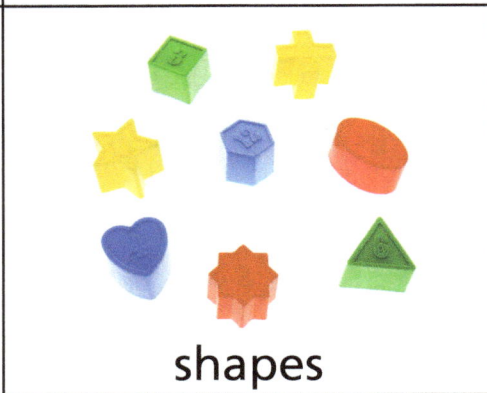 shapes	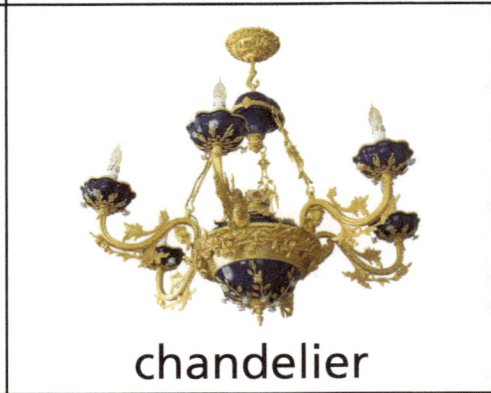 chandelier

Name _____

Helper Signature _____

Speech - Language Pathologist _____

Date _____

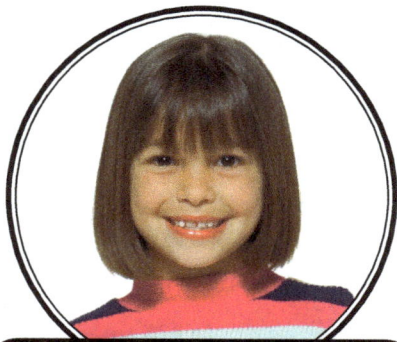

Sheila

This is Sheila. She shielded all the things on this page.

SH – Initial Position

1. Practice your sound by saying the words on this page. (Ex. shed, shears, etc.). Say the last word twice.

2. Practice saying **Sheila** with each of the words. (Ex. Sheila shed, Sheila shears, etc.). Say the last word pair twice.

3. Practice saying **shielded** with these words. (Ex. Sheila shielded the shed etc.). Say one of the sentences twice.

4. Practice saying **sheer** with these words. (Sheila shielded a sheer shed, etc.). Say one of the expanded sentences twice.

When you have finished this whole page you will have said your sound in 100 words! Good job!

shed	shears	sheet music
shelter	shepherd	chef
shaggy dog	sheets	sheriff

Name _____

Helper Signature _____

Speech - Language Pathologist _____

Date _____

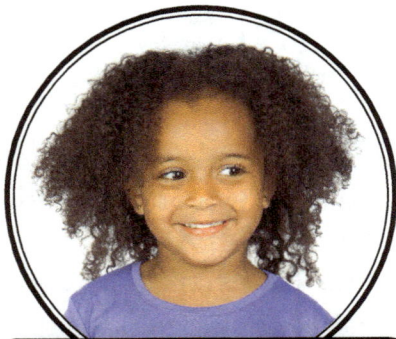

Shyla

This is Shyla. She shined all the things on this page.

SH – Initial Position

1. Practice your sound by saying the words on this page. (Ex. sheep, shin, etc.). Say the last word twice.

2. Practice saying **Shyla** with each of the words. (Ex. Shyla sheep, Shyla shin, etc.). Say the last word pair twice.

3. Practice saying **shined** with these words. (Ex. Shyla shined a sheep, etc.). Say one of the sentences twice.

4. Practice saying **shiny** with these words. (Shyla shined a shiny sheep, etc.). Say one of the expanded sentences twice.

When you have finished this whole page you will have said your sound in 100 words! Good job!

sheep	shin	shingle
ship	shirt	Chicago
shield	shipwreck	shallow pool

Name _____

Helper Signature _____

Speech - Language Pathologist _____

Date _____

#BKCD-273 • *Say & Do® Artic Reps* • ©2015 Super Duper® Publications • www.superduperinc.com

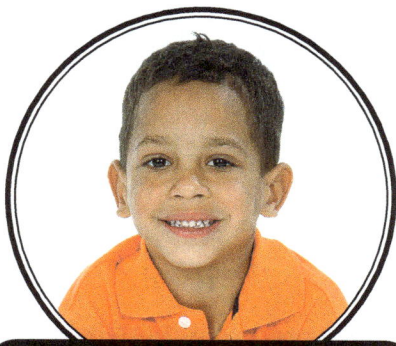

Shondel

This is Shondel. He showed all the things on this page.

1. Practice your sound by saying the words on this page. (Ex. shoe, shoppers, etc.). Say the last word twice.

2. Practice saying **Shondel** with each of the words. (Ex. Shondel shoe, Shondel shoppers, etc.). Say the last word pair twice.

3. Practice saying **showed** with these words. (Ex. Shondel showed the shoe, etc.). Say one of the sentences twice.

4. Practice saying **short** with these words. (Shondel showed a short shoe, etc.). Say one of the expanded sentences twice.

When you have finished this whole page you will have said your sound in 100 words! Good job!

shoe	shoppers	shave
chauffeur	shoemaker	shooting star
shopping cart	shopping mall	shore

Name

Helper Signature

Speech - Language Pathologist

Date

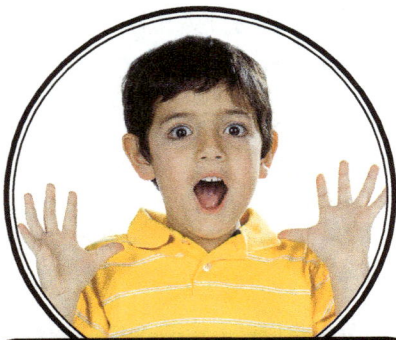

Shawn

This is Shawn. He shook all the things on this page.

SH - Initial Position

1. Practice your sound by saying the words on this page. (Ex. shotput, shoulder, etc.). Say the last word twice.

2. Practice saying **Shawn** with each of the words. (Ex. Shawn shotput, Shawn shoulder, etc.). Say the last word pair twice.

3. Practice saying **shook** with these words. (Ex. Shawn shook the shotput, etc.). Say one of the sentences twice.

4. Practice saying **sugary** with these words. (Shawn shook a sugary shotput, etc.). Say one of the expanded sentences twice.

When you have finished this whole page you will have said your sound in 100 words! Good job!

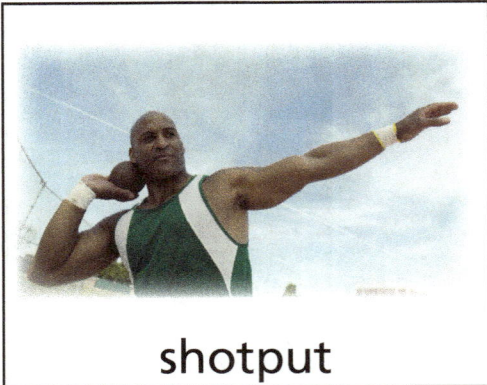 shotput	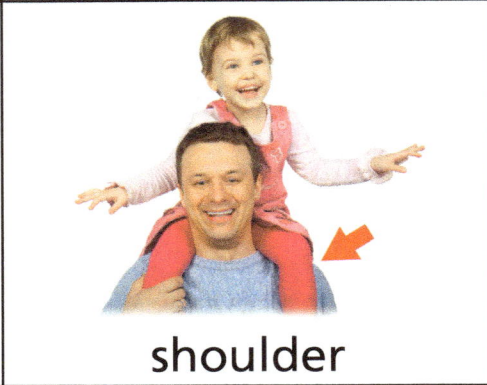 shoulder	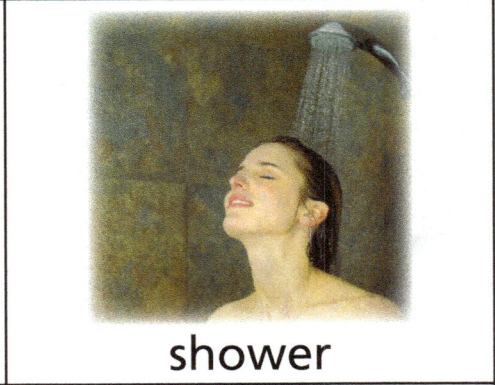 shower
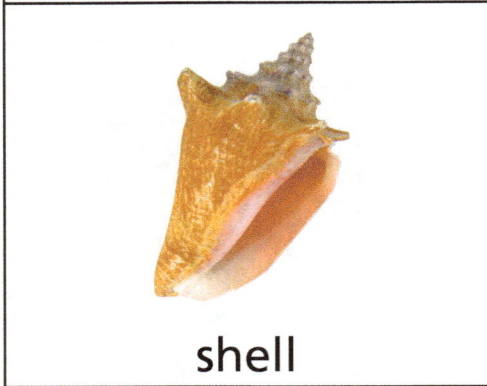 shell	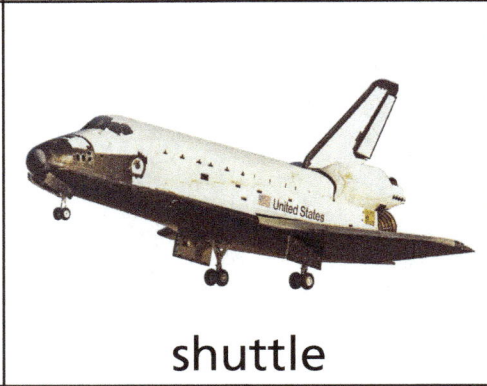 shuttle	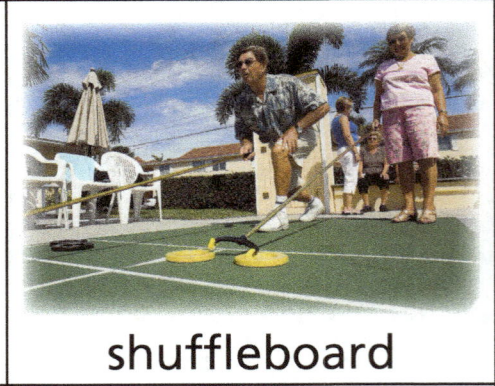 shuffleboard
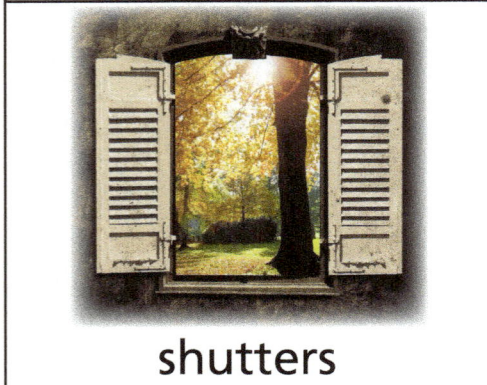 shutters	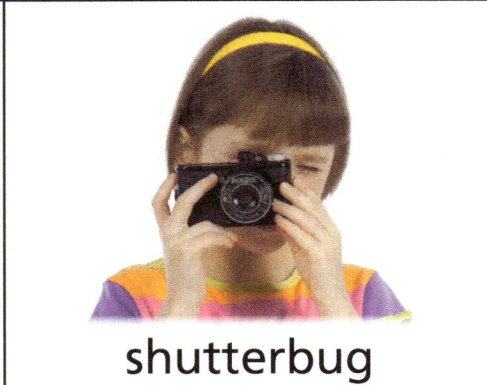 shutterbug	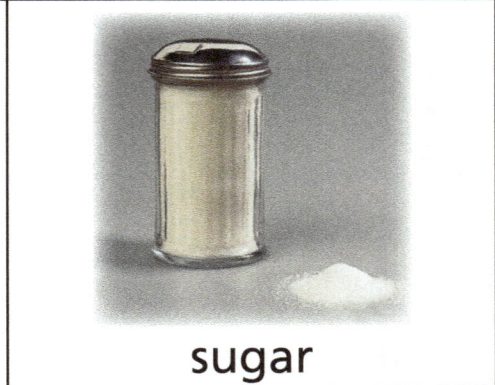 sugar

Name _____

Helper Signature _____

Speech - Language Pathologist _____

Date _____

#BKCD-273 • *Say & Do® Artic Reps* • ©2015 Super Duper® Publications • www.superduperinc.com

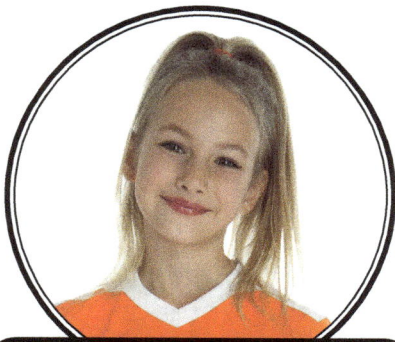

Ashley

This is Ashley. She was wishing for all the things on this page.

1. Practice your sound by saying the words on this page. (Ex. cashew, lotion, etc.). Say the last word twice.
2. Practice saying **Ashley** with each of the words. (Ex. Ashley cashew, Ashley lotion, etc.). Say the last word pair twice.
3. Practice saying **was wishing for** with these words. (Ex. Ashley was wishing for a cashew, etc.). Say one of the sentences twice.
4. Practice saying **delicious** with these words. (Ashley was wishing for a delicious cashew, etc.). Say one of the expanded sentences twice.

When you have finished this whole page you will have said your sound in 100 words! Good job!

cashew	lotion	wishbone
seashore	dishpan	tissue
marshmallow	parachute	milkshake

Name _____

Helper Signature _____

Speech - Language Pathologist _____

Date _____

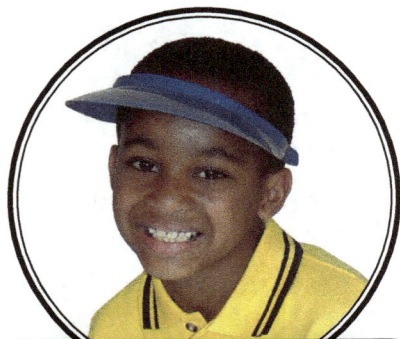

Rashid

This is Rashid. He was polishing all the things on this page.

SH – Medial Position

1. Practice your sound by saying the words on this page. (Ex. dish rack, fish tank, etc.). Say the last word twice.

2. Practice saying **Rashid** with each of the words. (Ex. Rashid dish rack, Rashid fish tank, etc.). Say the last word pair twice.

3. Practice saying **was polishing** with these words. (Ex. Rashid was polishing the dish rack, etc.). Say one of the sentences twice.

4. Practice saying **flashy** with these words. (Rashid was polishing a flashy dish rack, etc.). Say one of the expanded sentences twice.

When you have finished this whole page you will have said your sound in 100 words! Good job!

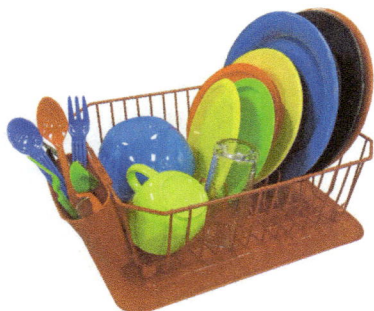 dish rack	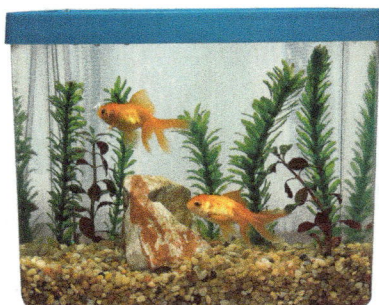 fish tank	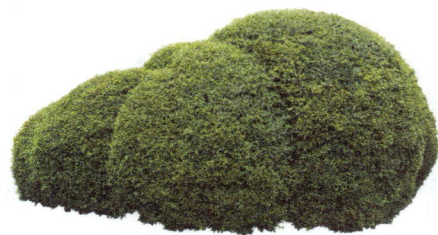 bushes
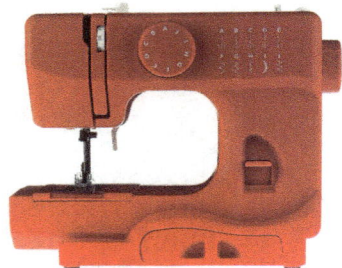 sewing machine	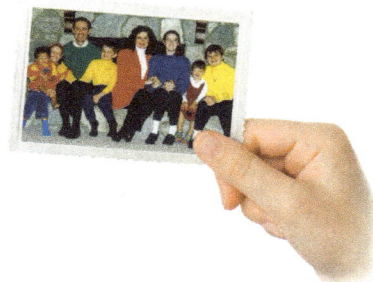 snapshot	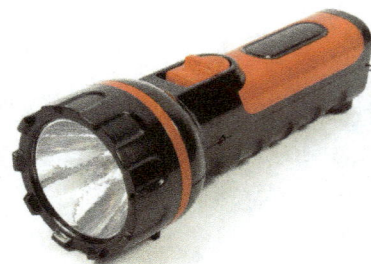 flashlight
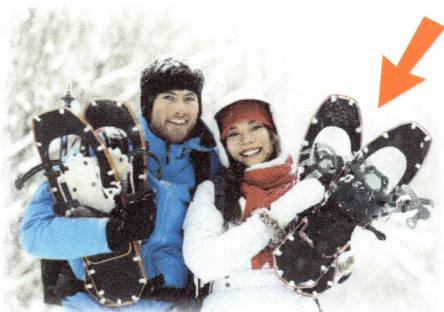 snowshoes	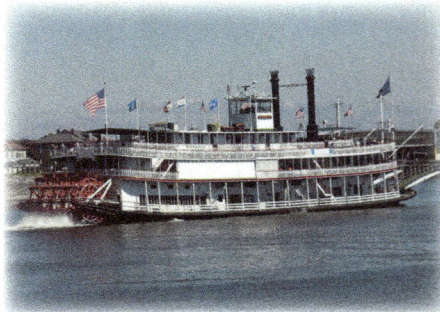 steamship	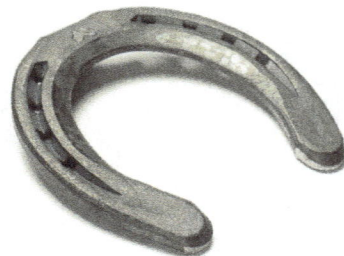 horseshoe

Name _____

Helper Signature _____

Speech - Language Pathologist _____

Date _____

#BKCD-273 • Say & Do® Artic Reps • ©2015 Super Duper® Publications • www.superduperinc.com

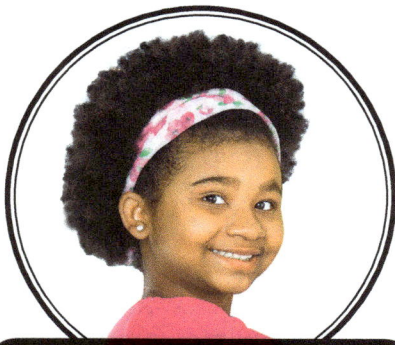

Latisha

This is Latisha. She was rushing to all the things on this page.

1. Practice your sound by saying the words on this page. (Ex. ocean, dishes, etc.). Say the last word twice.

2. Practice saying **Latisha** with each of the words. (Ex. Latisha ocean, Latisha dishes, etc.). Say the last word pair twice.

3. Practice saying **was rushing to** with these words. (Ex. Latisha was rushing to the ocean, etc.). Say one of the sentences twice.

4. Practice saying **special** with these words. (Latisha was rushing to a special ocean, etc.). Say one of the expanded sentences twice.

When you have finished this whole page you will have said your sound in 100 words! Good job!

ocean	dishes	wishing well
washtub	workshop	cashier
cushion	mushroom	glacier

Name _____

Helper Signature _____

Speech - Language Pathologist _____

Date _____

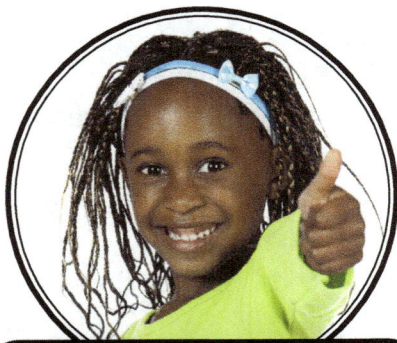

Tasha

This is Tasha. She was washing all the things on this page.

SH – Medial Position

1. Practice your sound by saying the words on this page. (Ex. mansion, gas station, etc.). Say the last word twice.
2. Practice saying **Tasha** with each of the words. (Ex. Tasha mansion, Tasha gas station, etc.). Say the last word pair twice.
3. Practice saying **was washing** with these words. (Ex. Tasha was washing the mansion, etc.). Say one of the sentences twice.
4. Practice saying **precious** with these words. (Tasha was washing a precious mansion, etc.). Say one of the expanded sentences twice.

When you have finished this whole page you will have said your sound in 100 words! Good job!

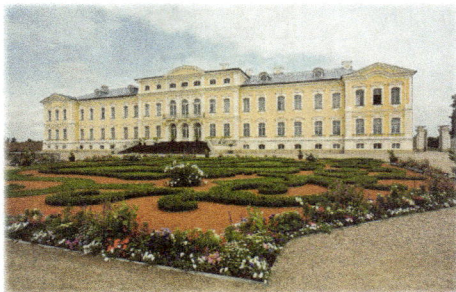	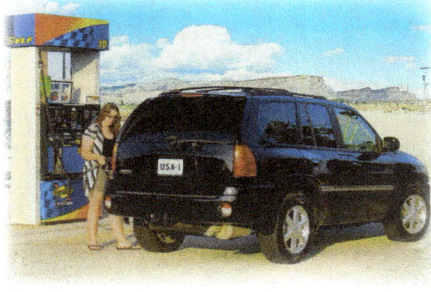	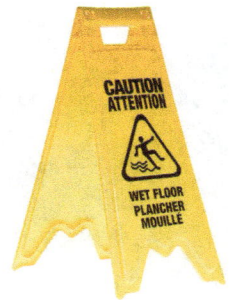
mansion	gas station	caution sign
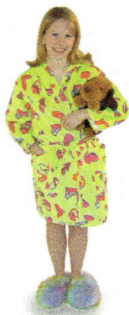	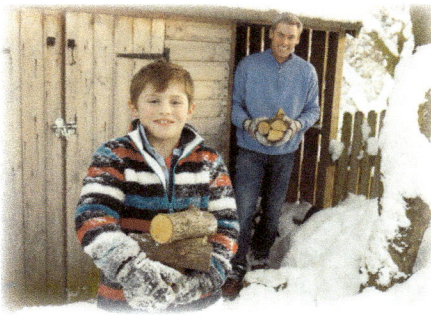	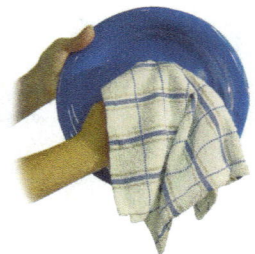
nightshirt	woodshed	dishrag
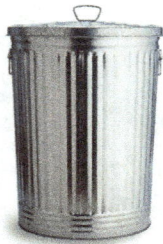	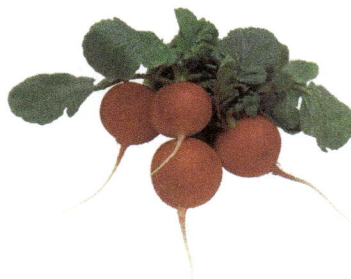	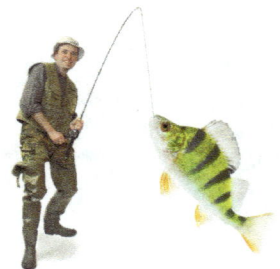
trash can	radishes	fisherman

Name _____

Helper Signature _____

Speech - Language Pathologist _____

Date _____

#BKCD-273 • *Say & Do® Artic Reps* • ©2015 Super Duper® Publications • www.superduperinc.com

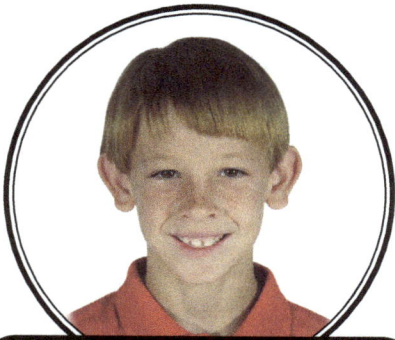

Nash

This is Nash. He will brush all the things on this page.

SH – Final Position

1. Practice your sound by saying the words on this page. (Ex. dish, paintbrush, etc.). Say the last word twice.

2. Practice saying **Nash** with each of the words. (Ex. Nash dish, Nash paintbrush, etc.). Say the last word pair twice.

3. Practice saying **will brush** with these words. (Ex. Nash will brush the dish, etc.). Say one of the sentences twice.

4. Practice saying **fresh** with these words. (Nash will brush a fresh dish, etc.). Say one of the expanded sentences twice.

When you have finished this whole page you will have said your sound in 100 words! Good job!

dish	paintbrush	fish
radish	hairbrush	mustache
blemish	ticklish	eyelash

Name _____

Speech - Language Pathologist _____

Helper Signature _____

Date _____

SH – Final Position

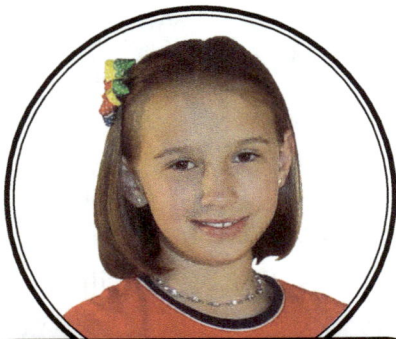

Trish

This is Trish. She can wish for all the things on this page.

1. Practice your sound by saying the words on this page. (Ex. nail polish, go fish, etc.). Say the last word twice.

2. Practice saying **Trish** with each of the words. (Ex. Trish nail polish, Trish go fish, etc.). Say the last word pair twice.

3. Practice saying **can wish for** with these words. (Ex. Trish can wish for nail polish, etc.). Say one of the sentences twice.

4. Practice saying **plush** with these words. (Trish can wish for plush nail polish, etc.). Say one of the expanded sentences twice.

When you have finished this whole page you will have said your sound in 100 words! Good job!

nail polish	Go Fish	finish
mouthwash	polish	crush
licorice	paint brush	relish

Name _____

Helper Signature _____

Speech - Language Pathologist _____

Date _____

#BKCD-273 • *Say & Do® Artic Reps* • ©2015 Super Duper® Publications • www.superduperinc.com

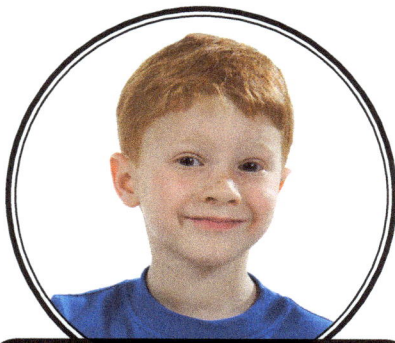

Josh

This is Josh. He can crush all the things on this page.

SH – Final Position

1. Practice your sound by saying the words on this page. (Ex. flash, wish, etc.). Say the last word twice.

2. Practice saying **Josh** with each of the words. (Ex. Josh flash, Josh wish, etc.). Say the last word pair twice.

3. Practice saying **can crush** with these words. (Ex. Josh can crush a flash, etc.). Say one of the sentences twice.

4. Practice saying **selfish** with these words. (Josh can crush a selfish flash, etc.). Say one of the expanded sentences twice.

When you have finished this whole page you will have said your sound in 100 words! Good job!

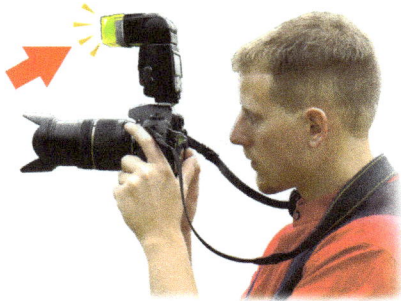 flash	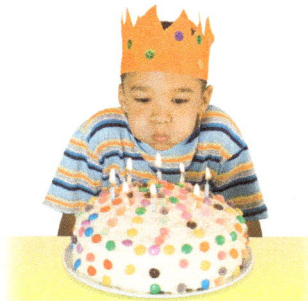 wish	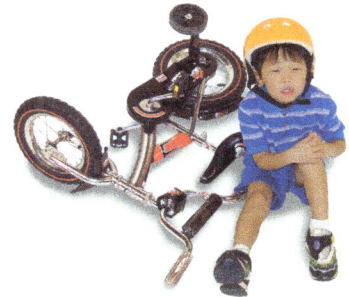 crash
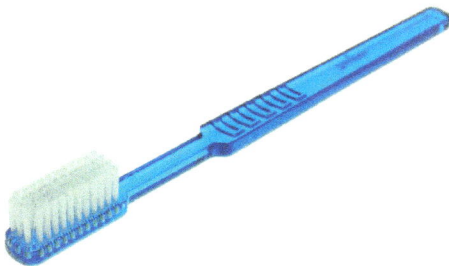 toothbrush	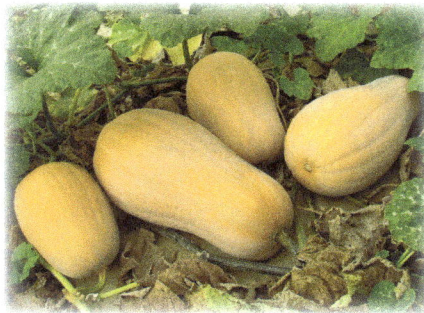 squash	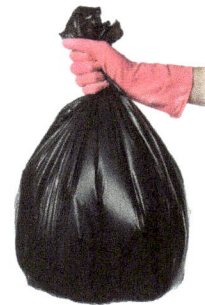 trash
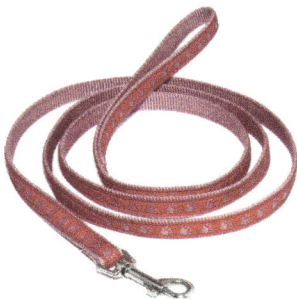 leash	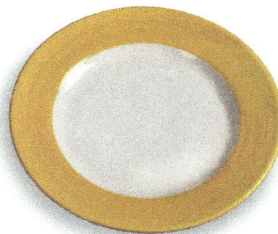 dish	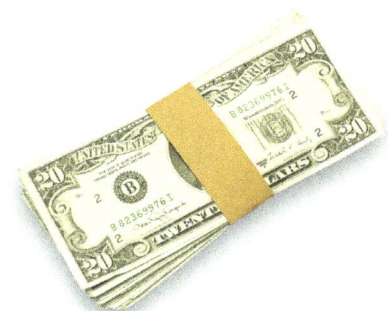 cash

Name _____

Helper Signature _____

Speech - Language Pathologist _____

Date _____

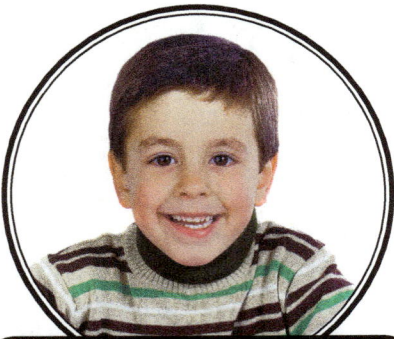

Marsh

This is Marsh. He can push all the things on this page.

SH – Final Position

1. Practice your sound by saying the words on this page. (Ex. catfish, rash, etc.). Say the last word twice.

2. Practice saying **Marsh** with each of the words. (Ex. Marsh catfish, Marsh rash, etc.). Say the last word pair twice.

3. Practice saying **can push** with these words. (Ex. Marsh can push the catfish, etc.). Say one of the sentences twice.

4. Practice saying **harsh** with these words. (Marsh can push a harsh catfish, etc.). Say one of the expanded sentences twice.

When you have finished this whole page you will have said your sound in 100 words! Good job!

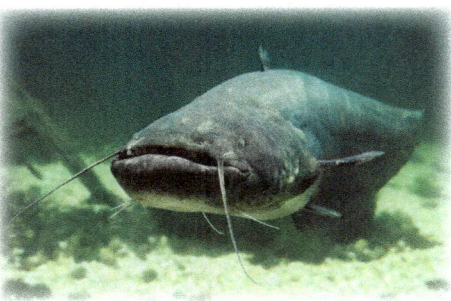 catfish	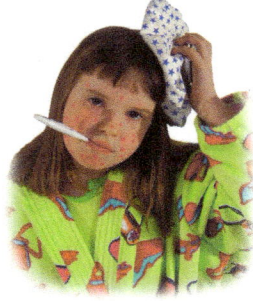 rash	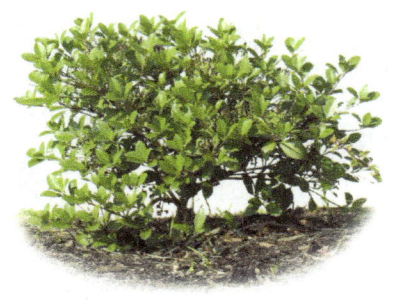 bush
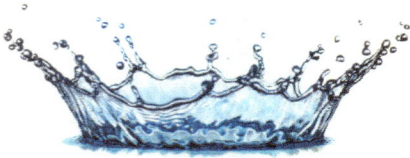 splash	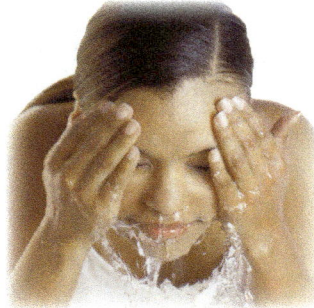 wash	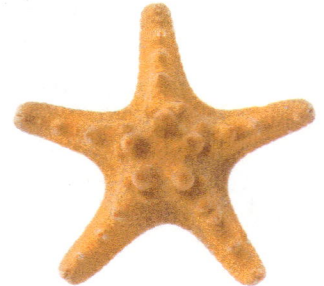 starfish
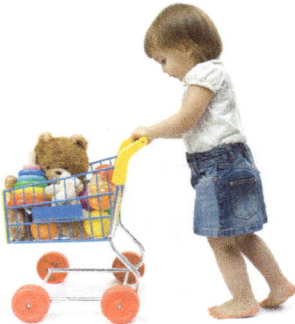 push	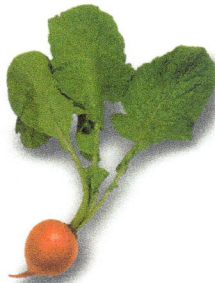 radish	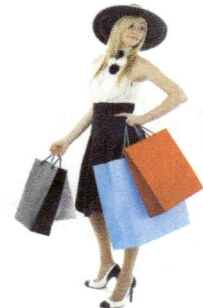 stylish

Name _____

Helper Signature _____

Speech - Language Pathologist _____

Date _____

#BKCD-273 • *Say & Do® Artic Reps* • ©2015 Super Duper® Publications • www.superduperinc.com